REFLECTIONS ON SPIRITUALITY AND HEALTH

STEPHEN G. WRIGHT FRCN MBE

ST MARTIN'S COLLEGE, CARLISLE
SACRED SPACE FOUNDATION

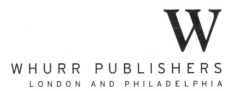

WHURR PUBLISHERS
LONDON AND PHILADELPHIA

© 2005 WHURR PUBLISHERS LTD

First published 2005
by Whurr Publishers Ltd
19b Compton Terrace
London N1 2UN, England and
325 Chestnut Street, Philadelphia PA 19106, USA

British Library Cataloguing in Publication Data

A catalogue record for this book
is available from the British Library.

ISBN 1 86156 468 6

Typeset by Adrian McLaughlin, a@microguides.net
Printed and bound in the UK by Athenæum Press Ltd, Gateshead, Tyne & Wear.

REFLECTIONS ON
SPIRITUALITY AND HEALTH

For Izzy, Zack and Martha

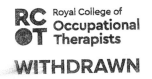

CONTENTS

FOREWORD

ON THE SURFACE

On the surface, it might seem odd that Steve Wright asked me to write the foreword for this book on *Reflections on Spirituality and Health*. He knows that I have avoided the use of the word 'spiritual' whenever I can in my work, since I am concerned it is a button-pressing word like 'God' or 'love', which can bar our communication – at least in a medical context. In the past I have argued with him that I would rather speak of the impact on our health of human caring, kindness, and connection – the everyday and universally recognised expressions of our communal search for meaning and wholeness, and our desire to care for others and make a difference in their lives. So why did I agree? Because the only thing that differs in our search is our vocabulary. Also, our dialogue and this book mirror the many dialogues in our culture that are striving to bridge the gaps we have created – of the technical from the human, of our science from our art, of our medicine from our world of inner meaning, of our own hearts from our heads, our emotions from our thoughts . . . I have to admit that if any word is to be asked to gather in its arms a number of the threads of that enquiry, thus building a bridge across these gaps, then the word 'spirituality' is a powerful contender, standing in partnership with words like healing, caring and holism. Perhaps you can think of better ones? This book will stimulate your thinking around this, it may press your buttons (a good thing if experienced mindfully), and it may open your eyes a little more; it may even express what you have always known in your work and life: the value of life and of caring enough to care. People count, you count and the human factor can even outweigh the technical in producing change in health care. Yet our humanity is getting harder to find in the algorithms of treatments and the protocols of procedures. In this book you will find reflections, research and review that will enrich your own enquiry.

The other reason I said yes is because of Steve Wright's personal integrity. Spirituality in today's world can become a business, a vehicle for control and delusion. I am, as you can sense, cautious around this (but not around helping people rediscover a spirited life). I have watched Professor Wright's work and know of the honesty that characterizes him, and his pioneering work in medicine and nursing. So when he has shown the courage to expand his enquiry and care beyond the narrow confines of these worlds, I, for one, am happy to listen carefully to what he has to say and teach. This has taken me into a friend-ship with him, and through this book you in turn may come to sense something of the remarkable individual behind it.

Finally, he has even succeeded in getting me to express some of my own thoughts in the language of spirituality – wonders will never cease. It was William James who said, in *The Varieties of Religious Experience*, that we are all separated on the surface but connected in the deep. Perhaps spirituality 'in the deep of us' is our common ground. One aspect of our connection, our com-mon ground, is our desire to be released from suffering and to help others to be so released.

Professor Wright explores health, wholeness, hale, healing, holism, holy – words that are connected in the deep, in the common root of the Germanic word 'hælan' – and these things perhaps draw water from the same well, as do creative change and spiritual transformation. It is a well largely untapped in the recent history of orthodox medicine. For five decades metaphors of war and the emphasis on disease not health, have dominated health care, with its 'med-ical model' of 'anti' drugs and external blocking interventions, leading to unsustainable increase in costs. This era was not predicated on self-responsibil-ity or care or nurturing of life, but on the power of the treatment and intervention . . . the hope was that the latter made the former redundant. Human factors have become undervalued in a technical age, and in turn so have people and emotional and spiritual welfare.

Now it's changing. The 'anti' is being balanced by the 'pro' and issues of life's innate capacity – driven from one end by the popular movement searching for complementary and alternative medicine and wellness enhancement; but para-doxically from the other by remarkable new research showing that the inner life of people is a major factor in their illness and health – with loneliness, despair, and anguish driving disease and mortality (the main risk factor for heart disease are not just factors like cholesterol or blood pressure, but hopelessness). Com-munity, meaning, peace of mind, true happiness are being shown to nurture health. This sewing of the head back on the body, in turn is reconnecting what many would call the spirit – and new sciences like psychoneuroimmunology and affective neuroscience chart the oneness of life and people.

This emerging realization of the central importance of inner life on health, a holistic medical view resisting fragmenting of the inner life from health, in turn is resulting in a better ear for people's cry for peace of mind and heart and wholeness. This leads people to common ground shared by the many spiritual and healing practices – and as it leads the individuals involved, so too their cultures.

Central to this is respect for life – much illness stems from its lack, and an awakening of respect and compassion for self and others will aid health and encourage a reconnection to caring and constructive values, and so action. Research is showing that the innate healing systems (formerly dismissed when it turned up in response to a placebo) are powerfully impacted towards being made whole by human caring, hope, faith, and meaning – our faith can make us whole. (A recent study showed that during brain scanning, patients with Parkinson's disease who were injected with a drug to release dopamine often released the chemical in their brain when injected with a placebo). These healing systems are affected by inner peace (with its impact on physiology – e.g. see *www.heartmath.com*) and by relationship and our impact on one another – it has been claimed, for example, that the heart tracing (ECG) of one person can be read in the brain wave (EEG) of another when touching or very close.

Traditional spiritual practices such as the developments of empathy and compassion are being shown to be vital active ingredients, even prerequisites, in effective health care – in the carer and the cared for they build wellness and happiness. Effective and efficient health care must now (re)take into account these core values, and these are widely discussed in this book.

Involvement in religion is known to be good for health, bringing increased life expectancy of up to 15 years, and reduced disease (unless it creates guilt, punishment or abandonment feelings). Prayer brings positive physiological as well as spiritual change, compassion wakens up the same (left pre-frontal cortex) centre in the brain as antidepressants, placebo, happiness and spontaneous or faith-based healing. Brain scans of Buddhist monks have shown exceptional levels of activation of this area of the brain – challenging the Western model of happiness being a fixed 'trait', and suggesting it may be a trainable skill – perhaps there could be a better way than antidepressants for some of the four million people in Britain taking these drugs. Forgiveness comes arguably more readily to churchgoers, second only to love in the values of most religions – and this is the stuff of health – there is growing convergence and synergy between health care and spirituality, and this book bears witness to that. The world needs as many pathways to this wisdom as possible… and a restoring of the ancient link between health care and spiritual values, a core aspect of this book, is one contribution. Christ's work and miracles embraced the sick, as did so many other great spiritual teachers, and for many people, health care is a vocation.

The reluctance to see spiritual care as part of health care is changing. Reluctance to see health care as part of spirituality is also changing. Health care can be predicated on the life-respecting and enhancing values that nurture spiritual awareness. Nurturing staff's welfare, as Professor Wright explores, is needed however.

All this converges at the moment of the medical meeting. It can be brutal or mechanical, or, it can become a therapeutic encounter that creates human contact as a vehicle for powerful transformative creative change. Health care workers share in people's lives at times of 'sacred losses' (as the Rev Bob Devenny calls them), and then afterwards, when spirit and heart are broken along with body – and into these spaces can flow the presence of loving kindness, communion and the living expression of healing – which can rekindle a spirited life.

DAVID REILLY FRCP MRCGP FFHOM
Consultant Physician, The Centre for Integrative Care,
Glasgow Homoeopathic Hospital

PREFACE

This book explores the connection between spirituality and health. I have been writing on, researching and exploring this theme now for almost twenty years. During this time I began to question a lot of assumptions in my life, found myself plunged into mystical experiences and sought ways to ground all this in my ordinary life. Much of this experience has been published in my various writings, not least my regular column in *Nursing Standard*. It has generated some interesting correspondence, both supportive and hostile, some of which I have drawn on for this book. To some extent, those who have written of their rock-solid views about God impress me. Part of me is somewhat awed by a capacity to live in such absolute certainty, not just of the existence of God, but of His (sic) precise nature. To some, this fixed being is loving and kind, to others an ever-present figure of fear and judgement.

Personally, I've never been able to subscribe to the latter view. The notion of the angry, elderly, bearded, punishing (usually male) deity who zaps you because you had sex with the wrong person, has always seemed more like a projection from that fearful part of our own egos than a universal divinity. God is very real to me, and while my experience is personal and immanent, it is also transcendent and beyond words. I have long since learned never to try and pin this stuff down in absolutes, for to do so loses the magnificence of its boundless possibility. Yet the Big Guy that many people seem to be so sure and afraid of pops up in religions right across the world; but considering the multiplicity of faiths, He is very much a minority sport – most people it seems don't have much time for Him.

I have had letters damning me because I refuse to accept a purely Christian (whatever that is, bearing in mind that there are over 3000 sects, at least, across the world who call themselves Christian) perspective in my writings. Others from a more atheistic persuasion have offered condemnation for raising a theo-centric spirituality at all. Throughout this text, I have sought to draw upon perspectives from different faiths and none, and I am informed by my training at the Interfaith Seminary that there are many ways, but one truth. Thus, whenever I have used the word 'God' in the text, I have tended to qualify it in ways that I hope readers from different perspectives will find accessible. Thus 'God', 'Goddess', 'the Absolute', 'Source of All', 'Ultimate Reality', 'Universal Consciousness', 'Highest Self', and so on are terms I have tended to use interchangeably. There is a wide continuum of views, from those whose Source is strictly God-centred to those for whom there is only this human reality and nothing else; from those who experience, know or believe in something ineffable, numinous and 'supernatural' to those who find consideration of anything other than the rational, biopsychosocial experience abhorrent or irrelevant. In later chapters I have addressed some of these perspectives, for what is natural or supernatural, rational or irrational, shifts according to the viewpoint we take.

For some people, spirituality is nothing to do with healthcare staff; for others, including myself, it is central. The chapters in this book explore some of these controversies, not only through the acknowledgement of research and other scholarly and objective sources, but also through much personal anecdote from my own story. In this I have sought to weave together the scholarly and authoritative with the real-life experience of spirituality. There is much to theorise about spirituality, and I have attended many conferences and read many papers where the intellectual debates were fascinating and fun. But in the end spirituality is about practice, the way we live our lives rooted in what has heart and meaning for us. So, much of this book is rooted in my own life and what has heart and meaning for me. I hope that in sharing it you will find inspiration, challenge, comfort, answers, questions, practical advice, serious wisdom and joyful irreverence. One of the things I have noticed about spiritual practice is that it can get very serious. Lightness and humour have their place too. The most holy people I know also have a cracking sense of humour.

Some of my best friends are atheists, and one recently commented, 'But does it have to be God?' Well, no it doesn't actually. There is no doubt that to huge numbers of people, an interventionist, omnipotent being is a hugely significant part of their lives to the very end. A growing body of research, which I will explore, suggests that people who have a spiritual practice and set of beliefs to live by, which might be called religiosity, tend to be healthier and happier than those who do not. But, as I will explore, there is little evidence that the atheist is any worse off in this respect than the theist. What seems to matter is that we live our lives believing in *something*. I sat with someone who was dying recently and she smiled pretty much all the way through it, being absolutely sure that she was 'going home to God'. In comparison, another woman I was nursing was in terror of her impending end because of some past grave sin for which she felt she was going to have to account. Likewise, I have perfectly happy and healthy atheist friends who are content with the view that 'this is all there is' and feel they need nothing more. Indeed some suggest that having a belief in god/s can be seen as almost pathological, as I will explore – an aberration of the mind brought about by distorted views of the real human condition or feelings of low self-esteem or some other ego problem. Conversely, the religious have argued that those who are agnostic or atheist are avoiding the difficult challenge of exploring and relating to the possibility of something, God, an absolute that is beyond the personal, the ordinarily human.

A psychiatrist I met recently clung vehemently to the pathology point of view. He made me laugh (which annoyed him intensely!) for it seemed to me he had merely replaced one set of gods with another – in rejecting a divinity he worshipped his own certainty. In the core of all religions and belief systems is a mystical tradition that unites them all – from the Buddha to the Tao, from the Sufis to the Desert Fathers, from Jung to Eliot. At the core lies a recognition that any name for that which is ultimately nameless is but a reduction of the ineffable something (no-thing!). There is a running thread in all these of some sort of universal consciousness, an ultimate reality, a loving is-ness that binds all into one that has many names and is also nameless.

The problem with the mystic approach is that when we try to ground it, make it solid, provide a structure, code the beliefs and so on we run the risk of using the safe container not as a womb to birth the spirit, but as an instrument of social control. For many people, anything religious or mystical is simply not true. For them, this is 'all there is'. Human beings end at their skin and there is no reality but this one. That is not my experience, and I trust my experience, for I would never be content with faith. I am not interested in belief. What counts to me is knowing, and a knowing that comes from tried and tested experience through my spiritual practice. However, I respect the contrary views of the atheist and have no desire to convince people otherwise, so I hope this text will be accessible to all people of spirit – those looking to continue deepening their quest for understanding of what it's all about. The atheist or theist carer is equally spiritual. They just believe and express those beliefs differently. The same goes for patients, so all of us in health care have to be able to respond with spiritual support across the vast spectrum of human spirituality without judgementalism or proselytising. And that can be tough sometimes, especially when we encounter the darker evidence of fundamentalism and control, or our own deeply held beliefs are challenged by the patient's needs. However, through our capacity to embrace the continuum of spirituality, those of us who work in healthcare can offer a better service to those in need. Whatever way we view spirituality (and, as I shall argue, everybody is spiritual), whether theistically or atheistically, spirituality has moved human consciousness and health since we first etched those earliest cave paintings, since the first maternal and paternal instincts arose, or since the shaman's first journey into the spirit world in search of healing.

In the run-up to the 2003 Iraq war the Prime Minister addressed the nation. He left out the phrase 'God bless you' (unlike the US President) at the end, on the advice of his officials. Publicly suggesting a belief in a deity is still dodgy territory for our politicians. Keeping politics secular has been a tough battle, not least in remembrance of the religiously initiated strife of the past, whether wars or oppressions of other faiths.

Health care is just the same, even though many of the founders and pioneers of modern health care were often deeply religious people, such as Florence Nightingale. Fears of prejudice and bigotry creeping in have long held back the exploration of religion and spirituality in our health systems. This is accentuated by the dominance of the humanistic and rationalist paradigm in modern health care – everything must be approached objectively and scientifically. Fine when it comes to safe drugs – if I pop an artery today I'd like to think the nurses and doctors at the Cumberland Infirmary are clued up about the substances it's safe to pump into my body with knowledge based on sound research. But the illness experience is not resolved solely through science; much of being human is essentially unscientific, deeply personal and very subjective. This is the nature of what has meaning and purpose for us in our lives – the very essence of spirituality.

My friend (let's just call him Mac, not his real name) has a long and turbulent history of violence, prison, drug abuse and addiction of all sorts. He's had 15 years being 'clean'. In a recent meeting with the various members of his therapy team, they expressed astonishment that he has held it together so well and without a single relapse. And there had been many tough moments down the years when the bottle or the pills would have been a blessed, if temporary, release. Of his resilience, they asked, 'What do you put it down to?' His reply was simple and direct: 'A higher power. God, if you must.' Mac has had many conversations with God down the years and I have been honoured sometimes to be witness to them. The professional therapy team treated his response with varying degrees of embarrassment, condescension and in one case even a touch of hostility.

Mac was rather pleased with himself, acknowledging the courage it had taken to speak his truth for the first time even though he suspected, and was proved right, that what he had to say was simply 'off the map' as far as the team were concerned. So where are these research-based professionals who seem to be turning a blind eye to the evidence that stares right at them? An enormous volume of research now points to the significance of spirituality and religion to our health and wellbeing, as we shall explore. Mac has found in his God (which, or rather who, he has not been able to fit in any particular religion) a deeply personal relationship. It is the very basis of his being. It has allowed him to let go of all his addictions and come into a place that he calls being 'at home' in himself, a place of deep knowing of God through personal experience.

All kinds of things can go on in us when patients start owning up to God – many don't, simply because they fear the kind of response that Mac got. Our prejudices, fears, old wounds around religion, our inclination towards humanistic/scientific health care or whatever – these and factors like them serve to block out a whole dimension of the patients' and our own experience. Professionals such as nurses and doctors often lay claim to being holistic carers. How can this be so when we pull back from something that is of profound significance to huge numbers of patients? When we have nothing, if anything, to offer when patients encounter spiritual crises, except to hand them over to the nearest chaplain?

It is difficult territory, fraught with pitfalls. But tell me which bit of health care has *not* been, as we have pushed back the frontiers since its birth? Spirituality and religion matter and directly affect health – they are therefore worthy topics of study and practice for carers of all sorts. There is wariness of spirituality and acceptance of science in mainstream health care, but science and spirit do not have to be mutually exclusive, as I hope to demonstrate. And there has to be more to spiritual care than checking the religion and telling the chaplain.

Linda Thomas and Jean Gray at *Nursing Standard* had the initial idea to have a regular column on spirituality and health matters in the journal. For five years now my contributions to *Nursing Standard* have generated interest and controversy on a theme that is still full of much uncertainty for many nurses and other healthcare practitioners. These writings form the backbone of the material in this book, together with extracts from the editorials in the journal that I edit (formerly called *Sacred Space*, now *Spirituality and Health International*). With some recent updating, re-structuring and merging of related themes, it was clear, as Jean suggested, that this could all be worked into a series of chapters on themes where many practitioners have so many questions. I hope what follows answers some of those questions and, perhaps more importantly, contributes to the spiritual awareness that each of us requires if we are to provide spiritual support to those in need. For those of us involved in health care, I suspect our capacity to meet the need for spiritual support in times of suffering is directly proportional to the degree to which we have awakened and come to rest in our own spirituality.

There is more, far more, that professional carers can contribute here, not least because an exploration of spirituality would seem to be of direct benefit to ourselves as well as those we seek to serve.

Some have commented that all this talk about spirituality is just so much fluff, irrelevant to the hard-pressed world of modern health care. Immersed in the day-to-day pressures of caring, more staff, rather than more spirit, would seem a fair comment. With noses to the wheel and elbows to the grindstone, this is indeed a difficult position from which to look up and see how things might be.

Oscar Wilde wrote that 'We are all of us in the gutter, but some of us are looking at the stars'. I can't help feeling that patients might just get a better deal if a few more of us were stargazers.

REV. PROFESSOR STEPHEN G. WRIGHT FRCN MBE
Cumbria
September 2004

INTRODUCTION

Nurses will be familiar with Stephen Wright's work on spirituality through his regular column in *Nursing Standard*. Based on his own experiences as a nurse, counsellor and inter-faith minister, Stephen's articles provide information, support and challenge to all those health professionals who want to explore the spiritual dimension of their work.

There was a time when it would have been considered 'off-the-wall' to tackle these issues in a mainstream professional journal, but changing times coupled with Stephen Wright's unique style have produced a much valued source of knowledge and encouragement for staff and students working under pressure, but who are nonetheless keen to come to terms with their own and their clients' spiritual needs. It is groundbreaking work that goes way beyond the usual boundaries, written with freshness of ideas and style, and often a topical relevance. This is difficult territory, but Stephen Wright negotiates his way with a light steer, recognising the potential for humour amid the fear and trepidation.

Given the high level of thinking that goes into every article, and yet the accessibility of the writing, these pieces were crying out to be brought together in one volume. Each can be enjoyed as simply a good read or, equally, will be useful to those researching academic assignments in the area of spirituality and health. Some of the work has appeared in *Nursing Standard* over the past five years, but there is also new and expanded material, grouped together around major themes: the links between good physical health and the health of the spirit in a scientifically-dominated culture; the importance of attending to our spiritual needs in the workplace; burnout among healthcare workers; faith, belief and disbelief; the relationship between the 'carer' and the 'cared for'; and the spiritual journey. In pursuing these themes the author discusses topics as varied as death, sexuality, the role of TV soap operas in our lives; religion; fundamentalism, silence, power, love, meditation and much more.

Many healthcare workers enjoy an intimate and privileged relationship with other human beings; they are there at the crucial moments - from birth to death and everything else in between. Not surprisingly, there is a need for material that acknowledges the deep feelings and emotions that are at play in this relationship, for the space in which to explore both negative and positive thoughts and ideas. Without such acknowledgement and support, too many staff suffer burnout and leave behind a job they have loved. This volume offers staff and their managers a chance to open up some of these areas for genuine discussion.

JEAN GRAY
Editor
Nursing Standard

ACKNOWLEDGEMENTS

To Jeannie Sayre-Adams for being my loving spiritual midwife and adviser, nourisher and critic of me and this work; Ian for lovingly as always holding home together while I buried myself in the computer; dear friends Larry and Barbara Dossey for their encouragement to produce this book, Jean Gray for her editorial support at *Nursing Standard* and enabling these thoughts to come to light, and Ruth Williams and Chris Bowles, 'Perspectives' editors at *Nursing Standard*. My deep gratitude also goes to fellow students and teachers on the Interfaith Seminary programme, most especially my dear friend Miranda Holden. And to my beloved Pat and Canon Christopher Pilkington – she who fed me soul food and he who was as father to my spirit.

CHAPTER 1

IN THE SPIRIT OF GOOD HEALTH

Is that all there is
Is that all there is
If that's all there is, my friends,
then let's keep dancing
let's break out the booze
and have a ball
if that's all there is.

Peggy Lee, 1969

'IT'S NOTHING TO DO WITH US'

Getting fitted out with my uniform on the first day in nursing school (many more moons ago than I care to think about) was a rite of passage, an initiation into a new role, a new world of thinking, doing and being that was to be spread before me in the following three years of training. I guess that dates me – we called it training then, not education. And like most healthcare workers of my generation, the emphasis of learning was very much on practical skills and body physiology, with a hint here and there of psychology or sociology as a nod to 'total patient care'.

Somewhere along the line we got into a discussion about religion and the role of the carer. It came up, I think, for pretty much the one and only time for any depth of discussion as we got to the subject of 'last offices' – what you do with the body when somebody dies. Among the instructions to get the false teeth in right (indeed, to make sure they were the right false teeth and not somebody else's!), mark the name on the body in the correct places and make sure various tubes and orifices were properly sealed, was a consideration of the patient's faith. I say 'consideration', when really there was a list of instructions about the various taboos of the most common religions, and that was about it.

The patient was to leave my care with about as much attention to their religion as they came into it. Textbooks for our course were equally limited – a bit of advice at best around the do's and don'ts of different belief systems and that was about it.

And we got to know the patient's religion by asking them on admission. There was a little place reserved in the top right-hand corner of the notes where 'Jewish' or 'Muslim' or 'R/C' or 'C of E' could be written. Those who couldn't decide on their religion or did not have one somehow did not fit the rules, so they usually got labelled 'C of E' just to make things tidy! And thus the record was complete, but largely ignored by all except the chaplains of various denominations who would visit to check which patients were 'theirs', or there would be a flurry of attention to it by everyone if death were looming. And that was about it. Spiritual care (or rather religious care, we didn't use the word 'spiritual') made easy.

As a pushy student I asked a tutor once, 'Is that it? Supposing the patient is worried about dying? Supposing they ask for a prayer or something? Supposing they want to know why all this sickness is happening?' My tutor looked at me with the look you might give the sole of your shoe when you stepped in something unpleasant on the pavement. 'That's religion, Nurse Wright, just pass the matter on to the chaplain. It's nothing to do with us.'

Learning about religion and spirituality in this way was the common experience of nurses and other healthcare workers of my generation. Times have changed. Spirituality has come out of the closet of ignorance. Now debates, conferences and publications on the issue are commonplace. The shelves of book shops groan under the weight of New Age and not so New Age texts giving advice on spiritual matters – everything from how to get your home more spiritual with Feng Shui to transforming your life through 'past life' exploration.

There is growing evidence that a major cultural shift towards matters spiritual is taking place, in Western cultures at least (Ray, 1996; Thomas, 1999). This means that increasingly patients place different demands and expectations of spiritual care in the hands of their professional carers. It also means that we are part of it too, for the doctor, nurse and therapist of whatever label is likely to be just as much part of this cultural shift as anybody else. So, like it or not, we are going to have to pay a little more attention to spirituality than hitherto, because it directly impacts upon healthcare theory and practice.

RELIGION AND SPIRITUALITY . . . IS THERE A DIFFERENCE?

Everybody seeks meaning, purpose, direction and connection in life. We all, at some point, ask questions on what it's all about, seeking answers to all those great existential questions like 'Who am I?', 'Why am I here?', 'Where am I going?' and 'How do I get there?' We all pursue relationships, work and activities that nurture and feel 'right' to us. For some people this pursuit is essentially god- or goddess-centred, embracing a belief in some divine being(s). For others, it is essentially atheistic or at least agnostic, as in humanism or Buddhism. Our spirituality is therefore the very roots of our being – who we think we are, why we are here and what we should do with our lives. Religion can be seen as the ritual, liturgy, dogma and the various practices that we collectively bring to our spiritual life to codify and unify it with others. Indeed some, if not most, religions provide ready-made answers to those questions we ask about the nature of our being and purpose. Religion provides a channel for the expression of our spirituality. Spirituality is the solid centre in our lives that enables us to express ourselves in the world and to cope with all the complexities and conflicts of being alive. Without it we can feel cast adrift, rootless, despairing and aimless, as Peggy Lee sang. Thus, everybody is spiritual, but not everybody is religious. We all seek meaning, purpose, relationship and connectedness in life, but not everybody chooses to channel that quest through the more formal structure and belief system of a religion.

Spirituality is about 'tuning the spirit within us to its source' (Kelting, 1995), about expressing our desire to be attuned as we 'hunger for a sense of purpose, destiny and value, grounded not only in ourselves, but in the wider nature of things. We also seek comfort and love, not just for and from one another, but for and from the greater realm of being.' Religion concerns 'rules and regulations, systems and hierarchies, the order of succession and the perpetuation of the religious institution. Ultimately it is about power', while spirituality is about 'personal, individual, intense, and often secret experiences of the presence of G-d' (Hartmann, 1997). Spirituality can be seen as that 'which inspires in one the desire to transcend the realm of the material' (O'Brien, 1982). Dr Lauren Artress, canon of Grace Cathedral in San Francisco, who has done much to restore the use of labyrinths as a spiritual tool, sees spirituality as the 'inward activity of growth and maturation that happens in each of us'. Religion on the other hand is 'the outward form, the "container", specifically the liturgy and all the acts of worship that teach, praise, and give thanks to God.' (Artress, 1995). It is interesting to note this concept of the 'container'. Religion is empty without the spiritual content.

Religion and spirituality are thus intertwined and for many the difference is meaningless, religion having provided a focus for spiritual expression and created the context for spirituality to emerge. However, the union is not always a happy one. Most religions have, historically, sought at some point to suppress any individual expression of spirituality, which challenges accepted dogma. In addition, others approaching from a humanistic perspective (e.g. Storr, 1996) have dismissed the religious and spiritual pursuit as a psychiatric phenomenon, a search for security and a father or authority figure in a difficult world. Meanwhile Nietzsche (1974; translated by Kaufmann), having famously declared that 'God is dead', saw the loss of belief as a great opportunity to voyage on the 'open sea' of humanity without the restraint of religious dogma. Humanism, the belief in the essential value and power of every human being without recourse to anything 'supernatural', was in part a reaction to religious orthodoxy and fundamentalism. But is there a risk that, as human values tend to shift with time and circumstance, moral relativism emerges, as can be witnessed in the debates which rage over euthanasia, abortion, genetic screening and so on?

Thus while spirituality for most people embraces some form of deity or transcendent realm, this is not a universal requirement. What seems to matter for our health and wellbeing in the world is that we believe in something – the goodness (or otherwise) of humanity, science, football or whatever. Whatever it takes to make us feel purposeful and connected in the world impacts upon our health. For most people, as we shall see, this does include some form of Absolute, God(s)/Goddess(es), Source of All or whatever name(s) they are given. However, spirituality also includes beliefs that are not theocentric. I have a dear friend who is an atheist, humanist and socialist, but this does not mean she is not spiritual, indeed quite the reverse. Her beliefs profoundly influence the way she is in the world, how she relates to others, her commitment to improving health care, how she supports her family and her community, and so on. Therefore spirituality may or may not be god-centred.

When we have a health problem, we may also experience a spiritual problem. Our illness story may challenge the way we look at the world. Fears of death, loss and injury can arise. Relationships can be shaken, hopes changed, expectations adjusted. Indeed, what we feel and believe about our health can directly affect it; there is a direct impact upon our cellular structure from our emotional state (Pert, 1997). We therefore need to look more deeply at spirituality because it directly affects the wellbeing of patients. This in turn challenges us to find more rigorous assessment tools and more appropriate ways of addressing people's spiritual needs than ticking the religion box in the case notes (Engel et al., 2000; Burkhardt & Jacobsen, 2000; see also Chapter 23). Furthermore, there is a growing body of evidence that stress, burnout and the disenchantment of professional carers with their work has its roots in issues more complex than pay and conditions. Issues such as meaning, purpose, relationships and connectedness in work (the very stuff of spirituality) are just as important as other matters, if not more so, in producing a happy and contented workforce and an organisation that does its job well (Snow & Willard, 1989; Goleman, 1995; Hatfield, 1999; see also Chapter 2).

Thus we need to look at more imaginative ways than hitherto of giving spiritual support at work to carers as well as patients. From the evidence available, it seems that relying on the chaplain alone is a hopelessly reduced way of looking at it. In subsequent chapters, we will explore in a little more detail some of the issues raised above and look at what might be useful to us from within and beyond the world of health care.

Scientific but soulless

Much of modern health care seems to have lost a sense of the sacred; technically and scientifically rich, yet spiritually poor. However, historically, it is deeply rooted in religious traditions. All the great faiths have demanded of their followers that they help and heal the sick, the poor and the needy. Many forms of religious orders and communities have provided care in various forms of institution, which evolved down the centuries into modern hospitals and clinics. Many of the great founders of modern professional care, such as Nightingale or Pasteur, were also deeply religious people who saw their work as a sacred act. The 'women healers' with their wisdom in the lore of herbs and birthing were often the only form of health care in many societies for generations (Achterberg, 1990). Indeed, it is these traditional ways of looking at and practising health care that prevail in many parts of the world – the modern high-tech approach we associate with Western culture is not universally available or accepted by all.

The high-tech, rational, scientific approach in modern health care has come at a price. Staff complain of often inhospitable environments and organisations, where disconnection and lack of meaningful relationships between colleagues and patients abound, where there is a seeming lack of reverence for life and human needs in the face of cost controls, workload pressures and the relentless demand to always act rationally and scientifically. In such a context, the spiritual needs of carers and cared for can expect scant attention. Despite the burgeoning interest in spiritual matters in the last few decades, in part demonstrated in the 'New Age' movement, spirituality remains very much within the realms of the luxurious add-on, something we might consider if we only had the time or when other priorities such as getting through the 'real work' (the drugs, the treatments, the therapies, the procedures) have been completed. Alternatively it is consigned to the realms of the personal and taboo – something that is not discussed or acted out publicly, lest we be seen as judgmental, fundamentalist or frankly flaky.

The oppressive history of some religions gives atheists grounds for concern, while religionists point to the atrocities done in the name of secular beliefs. Some of this concern spills over into the studies on religiosity. On balance, as Dossey (cited in Harrison, 2003) summarises, people who follow some sort of spiritual path in their lives live on average 7 to 15 years longer than those who do not. However, some authors have expressed concern that the studies that show such positive benefits (for good summaries see Dossey, 1999, Benn 2000) can be distorted by religious pressure groups to force more religion into health care (Sloan et al., 1999). Christina Puchalski (2004), head of the George

Washington Institute for Spirituality and Health, observes that Sloan and others are trying to 'offer a critique of those who do research into spirituality, health and religion, and I think rightly so'. She believes that:

> When you do the research and you say that people who go to church live longer, that's an association that arises when you look at a lot of factors. There seems to be some correlation with church attendance and living longer. It's an association of cause and effect, but there's also an association from a study showing that the people who attend cultural events live longer. So what does that really mean?

She suggests that some researchers may be trying to say 'Look that means you should go to church and you will live longer!', but in her view to suggest 'You should go to church therefore you will live longer' is too big a jump. Sloan and others are concerned that spirituality and religion are too private an area for physicians and other healthcare staff who have little experience to get involved. Certainly none of the studies are conclusive that a belief in God alone will make you healthy. What seems to matter is that you believe in something – enough to give your life meaning, purpose and connection.

Some settings seem to be successfully integrating spirituality and health without the risk of falling into bigotry and dogma, such as the Bristol Cancer Help Centre and the Glasgow Homeopathic Hospital. Spirituality in relation to the needs of both staff and patients are being integrated into everyday practice in settings like these (Wright, 2004a; Wright, 2004b). In addition, there has been some tentative attention at government level (e.g. Department of Health, 2004; NHS Scotland, 2002) to explore and support better ways of providing spiritual care (see Chapter 23). But these inroads have yet to encroach upon the great body politic of our healthcare systems. We have built the work of most caring professions ever more on scientific foundations, reinforced by what today is called 'evidence-based practice'. Florence Nightingale is often cited as a noble example of basing work on evidence – from her comments on nursing to recommendations for new sewers. She had mastered the skill of argument based on sound research, but this did not lead her to deny the inspiration for her work – an inspiration that defies scientific explanation – her mysticism and her belief that she was guided by God (B Dossey, 1999). It is worth remembering, as suggested above, that spirituality does not require a belief in God. People who work and believe in the values and practices of, for example, a state-funded health service are acting out their values based on their beliefs. Indeed it could be argued that the NHS is itself a spiritual expression – a practical application of a set of values concerning social cohesion, welfare and equality of provision. I suspect that a returning Jesus, Prophet or Buddha would not be averse to its founding principles. Furthermore, as we shall see, it can be argued that caring work is itself a spiritual practice (see Chapter 24). Despite the dominance of the rationalist, scientific paradigm in much of modern healthcare literature, education and practice, certain spiritual values and practices seem to have been retained. Indeed, if spirituality concerns 'right relationship' – relationship that has meaning and nurturance for us with ourselves, each other, the world and perhaps our God, and which is acted out in compassionate ways in the world – then most carers are 'de facto' being spiritual. Some people may pray, attend church or temple, meditate, commune with nature or do whatever is their custom to connect with the greater realm of being. Those working in health care have the advantage that the work being done is an equally valid spiritual practice – though we may often not recognise it.

Spirituality is not just a theory, it is a practice. Such practice is not just confined to our daily rituals or the pursuit of enlightenment. It is in our every waking moment, in the ordinary actions of life as well as the extraordinary. Caring and healing work is prescribed for followers of almost every faith. To Christians it is to love thy neighbour, in Islam to be merciful, in Buddhism to act compassionately, in humanism it is to respect and uphold the rights of others and so on. While every healthcare worker may not embrace the formal practices of a specific religion, each of us nevertheless has a spiritual discipline right under our noses – it is the work we do. Caring for others is a spiritual act.

However, we seem to have pushed spiritual values, whether god-centred or not, into the backwaters of healthcare consciousness. In our efforts to be non-judgemental and avoid bigotry and intolerance, we may also have created health services so focused on the mundane aspects of throughput that we have created a production-line concept of care devoid of meaning and purpose, the very essence of spirituality. Without attention to spirituality, to our lived experience of health care and what it means to us, whichever system we use to deliver health becomes dehumanised. Procedures replace relationality, policies replace connectedness and function replaces feeling. In such a reduced world, as the Reverend David Stoter (1995) suggests, 'to see spiritual care only as religious care limits its true nature and tends to relegate it to a footnote at the end of the ward report, or something to be handed on to another professional.' Spiritual care falls off the edge of our consciousness in our focus on the next target, the most efficient practice, the most cost-effective controls.

Paradoxically the rising interest in spiritual care and the possibility that it may even make health care more cost-effective (see Chapter 2) might set alarm bells ringing. Spiritual care might then become a new healthcare target with boxes to tick and quotas to be met, the very essence of what spirituality in health care is *not* about.

Science and spirit do not have to be incompatible and indeed, as this book will argue, a new alignment of the two, an integration as the examples at Bristol and Glasgow have shown, may produce even more benefits. Attention to spirituality in health care may indeed make it more, not less, effective. Some may fear that attention to spirituality, to what the humanist National Secular Society (Cobell, 2002) refers to as the 'supernatural', may lurch us back into a new Dark Age of irrational and dangerous health practices. It does not have to be so, as will be illustrated in many parts of this book. There is the possibility of a transcendent reality, of a realm of being, of a state of consciousness that does not necessarily fit with the currently dominant rational-scientific paradigm; such a state is not supernatural at all, but in fact deeply natural. Just because it is not easily measurable or quantifiable does not mean it is not there or that it is not important to people's health and wellbeing. The re-enchantment of health in a new alliance of science and spirit may be the launch pad for the greatest advances in health in the third millennium.

LOVE, LUST AND THE SPIRIT OF CARING

Many authors such as Alastair Campbell (1984) have described caring as a form of love, but not the love associated with affection, lust or attachment to things or persons. The compassionate concern and action for another's wellbeing, the love known as 'agape', underpins the loving, caring relationships that make healing possible in every interaction between carer and patient or client. Caring requires us to act with unconditional love for another in order to help and heal. Each time we reach out to comfort a crying child, hold the hand of a dying or suffering person or put in that bit of extra effort to make sure the patient gets what they need is an act of love. Whether standing up for the voiceless, the homeless and the disadvantaged, or arguing the case for the services someone needs, or making sure a treatment is given safely and painlessly, or struggling to meet the needs of the abusive or violent person (when we might be scared or trying to suppress our rejection of them), these take love. However, it is probably inadvisable to mention love, God or compassion in caring work – you may find yourself ignored, mocked or referred for a psychiatric opinion.

Without that loving connection to another human being it may be too easy to disconnect, dehumanise and see the other person as an 'it'. Buber (1937) considered two distinct ways in which we relate to others – the phenomena of 'I-It' and 'I-Thou'. When we consider something as an 'it', separation from us is implied. We cease to be in the right relationship with people, and come to see them as 'they' – 'things' other than ourselves. We have no loving connection to them, no relationality, no connectedness. What relationship there is, is one of dispassion, of commodification, of utilitarianism.

When we accept the essential value, sacredness, worthiness, and perhaps divinity, of the other, we relate to 'thou'. We love and care for and about them, not because they are different from us, or separate, or of use to us, but because they *are* us. We relate and connect to the other because we share a common humanity; in the other is ourselves, in ourselves is the other. What we do to them we do to ourselves for we are all connected, all part of each other. Such compassionate behaviour transcends person and situation, but is not necessarily an easy feat to achieve. It is relatively easy to find loving connection with the pleasant patient or the affectionate child, perhaps more difficult to find that same human connection with the mass murderer or child abuser.

The love known as agape enables us to bridge this gap, to make that connection. To be available with caring compassion for another is achievable because we do not see them as 'other', but as ourselves. Caring for our neighbour, no matter who we perceive them to be or what they have done, can be accomplished with equity and equanimity. When we see ourselves mirrored in the other, we are no longer separate. I become the patient. In caring for the other, I care also for myself. Yet, it is this transcendent quality of non-judgemental caring, whether explicit or not, that has underpinned caring ideals for centuries. Such caring love for another is an act of spirituality, a sacred thing in itself.

However, it must be remembered that there are risks for us when we attempt to give love, as the evidence of stress and burnout among carers makes clear (Williams et al., 1998; Health Education Authority, 1998; Borrill et al., 1998; Health and Safety Executive, 2004). Attempting to act with compassion and caring can leave us drained and burned out. Acting out roles ultimately depletes and disconnects us. When we pay attention to our spirituality and come to rest comfortably and deeply in our beliefs, then we can let go of the need to be in charge, the need to be in control, with all the inherent risks to us. Instead we can learn not so much to give compassion as to *be* it, indeed to be *in* it. From such a place, we are far less likely to exhaust ourselves trying to make it all work. But this way of being in the world rarely arrives by accident; it is the grist for the mill of our spiritual practice, as we shall see in later chapters.

Does such a view require us to accept the possibility that there is more than the brief flash of our existence in this world? That there is something greater within us and beyond us that brings meaning, understanding and compassion to the often nightmarishness of our work, which enables us to 'keep our hearts open in hell'? (Ram Dass & Gorman, 1990). If spirituality is about meaning, connection and purpose in the world, then belief systems that are not god-centred (humanism, Buddhism) would appear to be equally spiritual as those that are.

Darkness and light exist in all things. A humanistic perspective may teach us to seize the moment and ensure all our relationships are imbued with love and respect for others. If we end at our skin and there is no transcendence or transpersonal, and all we have is one brief lifetime, then we had better make the best of all the human relationships we can, protect this fragile planet for the next generation, and nurture, educate and respect others. However, if we acknowledge nothing beyond the merely human, nothing but our physical reality, no transcendence, are we left with only the strength of that 'self' to draw upon? Do we cast aside caring for others, if this is all there is, and exploit every-thing – people, resources and the planet? If this is all there is, is nihilism all that is left where it is simpler to take what you can and the devil take the rest?

Conversely, belief in a deity or deities as a focus of our spirituality is no guar-antee that we will act any better in the world. Some of the worst atrocities inflicted upon humanity, as well as grinding intolerance and illiberalism and the slow drip of indignity inflicted upon vulnerable people, have been done in the name of God – the gun in one hand, the holy book in the other.

THE CENTRE THAT HOLDS

In Western cultures especially, we worship at the altar of the rationalist, con-sumerist paradigm, the origin of which is largely attributed to the thinking of Descartes and those who followed him, where everything can be reduced to logic, quantity and observable evidence, and mind and body are separate. (Yet, paradoxically, Descartes was a devoutly religious man.) Jones (1996), a psy-chotherapist and professor of religious studies, believes that one consequence of the rationalist approach is lengthening queues for appointments with psy-chotherapists. Without belief in 'something other', a sense of the sacred, we suffer from disease and distress when life seems full of random events out of our control and no possibility of meaning and life exists beyond ordinary real-ity. One example of this is the impact upon current thinking in mental health care. As Barker and Buchanan-Barker (2004) have cogently argued:

> Contemporary psychiatry is typical of this materialistic world view, believing that mental illness is a function of chemical imbalance and that all so-called 'inner experience' is a mere by-product of brain activity. By focusing exclusively on the relationship between brain and behaviour, this view denies the importance of the spiritual dimensions of human nature and suggests that any such 'immeasurable' aspect of life does not actually exist.

Spirituality can transcend the limitations of human mind and body. It 'assures us that we are not alone', that 'we do not have to be in control of others' thereby allowing us to 'trust, to be honest and, therefore, vulnerable, and to live in acceptance of ourselves and others' and a 'faith in a power greater than ourselves' (Snow & Willard, 1989). For some people spirituality simply suggests a connection with the deeper meaning and purpose of life, and does not necessarily mean an acceptance of the divine. For others, coming home to a relationship with God, in whatever way the divine is perceived, is what a spir-itual journey is all about. The reduced world of 'just me and nothing else' may feed the need to be in control of everything, from the climate to the produc-tion of children. Jones (1996) goes on to note that fear of losing control seems to be one of the major symptoms of our age. 'Many an ulcer, hypertensive, or anxiety attack begins when contemporary men and women sense their lives slipping out of control' and this in turn lies at the root of many illnesses and a 'close-mindedness about spiritual experience'. Spirituality, and our deep hunger for connection and the sacred, seems to be fundamental to our sense of wellbeing. Perhaps we are also sick, dis-eased, when we are not in a state of complete wellbeing spiritually.

Thus the need to find purpose and meaning in life is not just a feature of those who are sick or close to death. It is a universal trait necessary for the maintenance of life and part of a well-developed personality. Conversely, anyone who has not deepened their understanding of their place in the scheme of things, who does not possess spiritual roots, may be seen as more prone to being diseased or unhealthy, and to risk inflicting this darkness upon others and the planet. Likewise, a carer who has not deepened understanding of their own spirituality is arguably less able to care for others in whom this need is present.

WB Yeats (Webb, 1991), in his poem 'The Second Coming', gives us a rich metaphor in the symbolism of falconer and falcon:

> Turning and turning in the widening gyre
> The falcon cannot hear the falconer;
> Things fall apart; the centre cannot hold;
> Mere anarchy is loosed upon the world . . .

The falcon is safe and secure, knows where it has come from and where to return while the falconer is at the centre of its circle of flight (gyre). Without the certainty of its centre, it becomes lost, cast adrift in the world, unsure of where to go, what to do.

Our spiritual core is like the falconer – calling us back to our centre, our home in a world full of confusion and disorientation, a place of security and certainty from which we can safely venture into the world. Time and again throughout the literature on spirituality we encounter this repeating theme: that spirituality is a kind of rock-hard centre within us, a place of solidity and certainty (or comfort with uncertainty), which holds us steady in a world full of complexity, paradox, extremes and grey areas. It provides map and compass, as well as the ship to guide us through life. Those embedded in such a world view seem better able to care for others, to be more available without judgementalism or the need to control, and better able to take care of themselves and their own health (Benson, 1996).

THE SPIRITUAL SUPERMARKET

The spiritual journey is not without risks, such as falling under the spell of cults and gurus or losing direction in the welter of options available in the modern-

day spiritual supermarket. Spiritual experiences can be profound and life transforming, but they can be interpreted by others as madness, especially when they
lead to behaviour that prevents us from being socially grounded and able to
function in the everyday world. There seems to be a great and growing hunger
for a spiritual connection in our culture, a hunger that the orthodox religions
often seem unable to satisfy. The pain of this hunger for the sacred in ourselves,
this existential angst, is then dulled by many with drink or drugs or serial relationships or spending, all of which fail to satisfy. As the effects wear off, we return
to face the very thing that we sought to escape, or lose the connection we
thought we had found while under their influence. Others need to withdraw
from the world for a while, but this can shatter relationships or lead to isolation.
In a recent speech in Manchester, the Dalai Lama reminded the audience that a
personal spiritual quest might or might not require a retreat *from* the physical
world for a time. However, it is quite a different quest when our intention is to
activate love and compassion for the purpose of relieving suffering *in* the world.

It is suggested in many opinion polls that Europe in general, and the UK in
particular, is still predominantly Christian. The majority of people, when asked,
describe themselves at least loosely as Christian. However, the exodus from our
churches continues unabated; vicars and priests regularly complain that they
only see their parishioners at births, marriages and funerals. Less than 2.5 per
cent of the population regularly attend church on Sunday, and the Bishop of
Oxford (cited in Storr, 1996) comments that 'We in Western Europe are now
in a post-Christian society.' Other religions appear to be capitalising to some
degree on this exodus, yet they too may have their problems in maintaining
membership and orthodoxy. Meanwhile a whole tranche of mixed and
matched cults and personal approaches, often loosely described as 'New Age',
is fuelling this decline. Perhaps part of the problem, as in health care, is the loss
of the spiritual tradition. Dogma, observance of form and ritual, obsession with
systems, structures and outcomes and the limited perspective of rational-scientific humanism sterilises the spiritual context. In the words of TS Eliot (1944),
we may 'have the experience, but miss the meaning'. If organised religions are
to survive, perhaps they will have to avoid the tendency to batten down the
hatches and demand orthodoxy, but instead find ways that embrace the burgeoning desire among huge numbers of people for individual spiritual
exploration and connection. Perhaps that experience of the personal and spiritual, bringing meaning and understanding to the work world, is what is
missing from health care as well.

Religion clearly still has a place; it is significant to many patients and carers,
the rituals and forms helping immensely through times of suffering. But is
there more to it than this? What about all of those for whom religion, where
it has become alienated from spirituality, ceases to have meaning or usefulness
or purpose?

Beyond unyielding despair

When care is not spiritual, it is dis-spirited. It contains the head but not the heart of caring and fails as a result. The outer manifestations of caring may be taking place, but something seems to be missing. It may be difficult to pin down and identify, and it may be that we know it by its absence rather than its presence. Patients especially are sensitive to it, though it may be difficult to articulate or make explicit. People can feel cared for, but not cared about. Carers go through the motions of caring, giving the injections, the sound advice, the hot bath, but some other dimension – conveying that the person is valued, loved even, is left out. Enough patients in the orthodox healthcare system seem to sense this, if the evidence from the escalating level of complaints and the seeking of alternative/complementary therapies and therapists are anything to go by.

Healthcare and social workers feel increasingly alienated in the workplace and often demonstrate this with their feet in the exodus from their professions. This alienation is not just the product of difficult workloads or poor pay. At a Spirituality and Health conference I helped to organise several years ago, one participant (an occupational therapist), close to tears, asked, 'How can I go back to that place when my heart and soul are not welcome there?' With so much of the work context bereft of a spiritual core, some try to integrate holistic practices and better relationships into their way of working, but it is often an uphill struggle. Others move on in the hope of finding or creating that safe sacred space in which their ideals can be fulfilled.

The picture is not all bleak; there are signs of change, although our health and social systems seem to be painfully slow in catching on. Industry, meanwhile, is rapidly learning that attending to the spiritual needs of employees is not only fashionable, but also cost-effective (see Chapter 2). Attention to spirituality in the workplace boosts profits and performance.

Recent thinking and research into physics, spirituality and psychology are pointing towards a new understanding of consciousness and energy, demonstrating an awesome unity and pattern in the universe, which is far from impersonal or neutral. However, much of this new thinking has failed so far to get through to our medical and nursing schools and teachers, many of whom remain hooked on reductionist biological, psychological or sociological models of human beings. Long ago Isaac Newton, regarded as one of the founders of the scientific age, yet also a deeply religious man, acknowledged that the more he understood the nature of things, the more he was convinced of a greater power and purpose that lay behind it – a phenomenon notable in the writings of other great scientists, from Einstein to Hawking. Thus perhaps we do not have to think in terms of science or spirituality, but science *and* spirituality. The new cosmology of the post-modern era seems to be embracing transpersonal phenomena, and a new model may thus be emerging. Ancient mysticism and quantum physics have much in common. What we may be doing is rediscovering an ancient model, to which modern science is now lending new credibility in a secular world. The notion of a universe where everything is interconnected and united, by the same force of energy as described by modern physics, would not be out of place in ancient spiritual texts or the view of any mystic.

This point is illustrated in the writings of Skolimowski (1992), philosopher and ecologist (ecophilosopher), from whose work the notion of ecopraxis has emerged. He is particularly scathing of modern philosophy, which is seen as having little to say about the wider world, the cosmos and our connection to it as human beings. For the carer, this means living and working in the world in ways that are 'sensitive to environments, to vibrational energy fields', and such carers see themselves 'as compassionate in relation to everything else'. This 'ecological person's' spirituality embraces sensitivities such as 'logic, intuition, morality, aesthetics and a sense of the sacred'. Being 'cocreators, we are capable of moving to a higher order in their (our) lives, guided by moral codes . . . ecophilosophy . . . depicts a view that is life-orientated, and about the inter-connectedness of all things, compassionately united with the flow of life in the universe'. Such a view of our place in the cosmos is echoed in thinking on spirituality both ancient and modern. From the Upanishads to Einstein, the notion of the interconnectedness of all things in the universe, ourselves included, pro-vides the ethical thrust for our compassionate concern for others, the world and ourselves. When we recognise our place in the awesome history of evo-lution and the cosmos, when we see ourselves as a strand in the web that connects us all, it is difficult not to be reverential to all of creation.

To the Native Americans, such a spiritual path is nothing new. The Navajo nation sees the spiritual path as 'walking the beauty way' – living in the grace of the wonder of the universe and being reverential for all of creation. A 'com-ing home' to our own spirituality, seeing ourselves as part of the whole, enables us to let go of so many of the 'ties that bind' and helps us facilitate the health of others, and in so doing to be healthy ourselves. Our health and that of oth-ers are intimately connected to our desire to be whole. It is not possible to be whole without the knowingness of our unique part in the whole.

Spirituality is thus fundamental to right relationships with ourselves, others and beyond. Without it, we live in a world bereft of heart and meaning. Schumacher (1977) notes:

> *A person, for instance, entirely fixed in the philosophy of materialistic scientism, denying the reality of the 'invisibles' and confining his attention solely to what can be counted, measured and weighed, lives in a very poor world, so poor that he will experience it as a meaningless wasteland unfit for human habitation. Equally, if he sees it as nothing but an accidental collocation of atoms he will needs agree with Bertrand Russell that the only rational attitude is one of 'unyielding despair'.*

In other words, part of the malaise in caring relationships may be an inner one, a loss of acceptance of the transcendent, the divine, to look both in and beyond ourselves or society for our moral guidance or codes of practice.

Right relationships begin with ourselves, but many spiritual traditions uphold that we cannot come to know ourselves without knowing God, the Absolute, our Highest Self, the Source of All, however we perceive that to be. The spiritual exploration may therefore inevitably transcend the very limited scientific view of what we are as human beings and cause us to re-examine and incorporate spiritual values into caring work. When this occurs, the healing potential explodes into many more possibilities. The hospital, clinic or nursing home, for example, could be revived as a place of short- or long-term retreat, nurturance, succour and healing, and turned away from the modernist, revolving-door, clinical, sickness machine that so many settings have become. New relationships can come into existence, which recognise the value of being with people as much as doing to them. Carers can let go of the intense effort required to give compassion, and relax into *being* compassionate, *being* healing. In short, we become the sacred space (Wright & Sayre-Adams, 2000) in which healing occurs. Spirituality and the sacred are illuminated in right relationships.

Mark Young (cited in Forder & Forder, 1995), an osteopath and follower of the Islamic Sufi tradition, has this to say:

> *There can be a moment in healing when there is perfect balance and all distinction . . . between healer and wounded disappears. It is at this point that something else can enter and both are transported to a place of mystery. Part of us yearns to return to this place, because it is here that we are made whole.*

When we enter into right relationships – characterised by connection, meaning, harmony, purpose, understanding and so on – not only with the world and each other, but also with ourselves and perhaps our God, then we find that place where we don't merely give healing, we become healing. The search for right relationship, with all that is – this is the essence of spirituality – and it is deeply connected to the wellbeing of ourselves and others and indeed of the whole of creation. Spirituality is part of health, not peripheral but core and central to it. It pervades our every thought and action, each caring moment. Spirituality and health are bonded to each other, inseparable companions in the dance of joy and sadness, health and illness, birth and death.

CHAPTER 2
SOUL WORKS – THE RELEVANCE OF SPIRITUALITY TO A HEALTHY WORKPLACE

They all attain perfection when they find joy in their work. Hear how a person attains perfection and finds joy in their work. A person attains perfection when their work is worship of God, from whom all things come and who is in all.

The Bhagavad Gita (translated by Mascaro, 1962)

A REFLECTIVE MOMENT

Conferencing can be hard going, especially if you are one of the speakers and the world and his mother seem to want to ask you a question, tell you you're wonderful or awful, or give you a lecture of their own. I found a quiet corner behind the coffee machine and watched the snow fall on the skylight. The hall was packed and noisy, but watching those flakes alight on glass and slowly melt I was overcome by a deep peacefulness. I felt utterly present, at home, just sitting and watching and strangely aware of the room and the people in it and everything that lay beyond it in a boundless whole. Nothing seemed separate, absolutely nothing. Everything was moving, and everything was perfectly still.

Such reveries, flashes of insight and moments of wordless wonder at the unity of all are common and part of the religious/spiritual experience that human beings encounter. Many studies, for example Hay and Hunt (2000) and MORI (2003), suggest that a belief in God and/or a mystical, spiritual and transcendent experience is still the norm for the majority of the population of the UK. This is borne out in other studies across the world, illuminating the international trend towards an increase in spiritual experiences and desire for them outside the formal structure of religion (e.g. an Australian survey by Tacey (2003) and a European-wide one by Lambert (cited by Hay, 2004)). Across the world, results vary according to the types of questions asked and how 'spiritual' is defined, but the overwhelming impression is that spirituality is part of the human make-up;

it is deeply embedded in the very essence of our being. The desire to relate is programmed into us, it seems, from the moment of birth as we seek a connection with our mother. David Hay (2004) at a recent conference in Aberdeen showed a stunning video of the work of Emese Nagy, at Dundee University, demonstrating how even tiny neonates mirrored the gestures of their mothers. And into adulthood we seek to know ourselves and that which is beyond the self. Some studies have borne out the possibility that we are indeed 'wired for God', such as that by Newberg et al. (2001) and Hamer (2004), who postulated an evolutionary cause. According to this view, the possibility of spirituality and religiosity has survival advantages. The argument goes that being alive and aware of death can be so terrifying that belief, for example in an afterlife or a loving universal power, enables human beings to cope with the world and survive it better than those who do not. Thus, down the long millennia, God got wired into our neurological pathways because we needed him/her/it there. That's one theory. Another of course is that the wiring is there because the One ordained it thus so that we could connect with an Ultimate Reality, the Absolute. In the first scenario, God or the Source of All is no more than a by-product of evolutionary processes, a mere figment of mental conjuring embedded in our genes to keep us safe. In the second the divine is very real and our whole make-up is geared to seeking that truth. However, Newberg et al. suggest further that:

> *While our neurological model offers a possible explanation of how we experience the mystical state of pure awareness, it proves nothing about the Absolute Unitary Being. It does not explain whether absolute being is nothing more than a brain state or, as mystics claim, the essence of what is most fundamentally real. Yet our work has convinced us that the mystics, at the very least, are not delusional or psychotic: they are certain beyond the shadow of a doubt that their experiences are real.*

To know that you are not judged psychotic for having a religious/spiritual event may come as something of a relief. Indeed, as many studies cited in the final chapter have shown, people who pay attention to meeting their spiritual needs tend to be healthier, happier and longer lived than those who do not. The interior mystical experience is indeed difficult to measure, simply because it is so personal and does not lend itself easily to the medium of words. Yet we can see exterior evidence of it, not just in the general wellbeing of the person but in the effects of their presence in the world. The mystical experience, unlike the psychotic, tends to have an expansive quality to it – the reverse of the psychotic. The mystic is more available, more loving, more creative, more compassionate, more committed to action for the wellbeing of others. Mysticism and the spiritual search are the foundations of the work of many great artists, philosophers, scientists and social activists from Nightingale to Einstein, from Marcus Aurelius to Gandhi, from TS Eliot to Walt Whitman.

The burgeoning interest in spirituality, and especially the hunt for an experience of it, is well documented, as some of the studies cited above have
suggested. Yet Western secularism has been pushing in the opposite direction.
If we are wired to tune to God (of some sort) what happens to our health if
we don't? James Jones (1996), a psychotherapist and professor of religious studies, has one response:

> *For the last two hundred years, Western culture has been an experiment to test the
> hypothesis that human beings can be totally fulfilled in an atmosphere of secular
> rationalism, technological efficiency, and material abundance alone. Evidence for the
> falsity of the claim that we live without meaning daily pours into the psychotherapists'
> offices. We see the anomie and emptiness symptomatic of the ethos with its disconnection
> from anything smacking of value, purpose, or the experience of the sacred.*

Spirituality – the search for wholeness, meaning, purpose and connection
and the resolution of those great existential questions that we explored in
Chapter 1 – is part of our very existence. Everyone searches at some level and
at some time for answers to questions about the meaning of life, thus everyone
is spiritual. And some choose to express that search through the more formal
'Here's an answer I've already prepared for you' path of some religions.
Nowhere do we find the search more apparent than in our work, whatever
form it takes; yet for huge numbers of people, work has become positively
unhealthy, un-wholing, devoid of meaning and purpose.

DISPIRITED WORK

'It's soulless,' he said, close to tears, 'completely soulless; how can I go back
there?' To find an executive of a well-known supermarket chain reduced to a
disempowered and miserable state on your floor is not the kind of image we
associate with the thrusting, reinvigorated economy of a prosperous Western
democracy. Of course, burned-out employees in the workplace are nothing
new. Neither is the experience of this young man who, when he ventured to
tell of his difficulties to his boss, found the victim getting the blame . . . 'There
must be something wrong with you that you can't take the pace.'

He'd gone through the usual corporate team bonding, goal setting, power
building, motivation groups at work. Everybody seemed caught up in the same
push for growth – more sales, more profits, more . . . The people become the
fodder for the sacred cow of profit. Working together as human beings?
Having life beyond work? Conversations beyond macho posturing and the latest female or football scores? All that stuff is for wimps. If you can't stand the
heat, stay out of the kitchen. Survival of the fittest (and that means the most
ruthless) is what counts, and there's no room for the human or the humane.

Resources are for better systems, leaner structures and more efficient and effective ways of working in order to make sure you stay in the lead. The game is about winning – and selling or achieving more and costing less is what wins. And it's not just aggressive capitalist companies that experience this malaise. Briskin (1998) suggests that any kind of work that is devoid of meaning is ultimately dispiriting and destructive, and has partly been fuelled by the industrial revolution, when work, which had hitherto been largely rural and in small units or self-directed agriculture, lost its relational quality. People no longer had control over their patterns of work but became caught up as cogs in a machine. And this seems to affect all work sectors. Whether commercial or public enterprises, small or large, charitable or profit making, there are variations in dis-ease, stress and burnout levels (and burnout, as Vaughan (1995) has pointed out, is always a spiritual crisis, not a psychological one; see Chapter 4) but they are variations on a theme – the overall picture is one of stressors at work producing astronomically high levels of dis-ease, disconnection and dissatisfaction (Health and Safety Executive, 2004; Health Education Authority, 1996; Confederation of British Industry, 1999).

There's an old joke about Tonto and the Lone Ranger, the heroes of a famous early TV western. Surrounded by hostile tribes, moving in for the kill, the Lone Ranger turns to Tonto and says, 'Well, looks like we've had it this time Tonto.' To which his faithful sidekick replies, 'What's this "we" business?'

Many people at work sometimes feel their relationships function like this. Relationships are not always as supportive as they might be. Many studies have illuminated how relationships at work are really power struggles rather than the collaborative efforts of supportive and egalitarian teams (e.g. see Hugman's (1991) work amongst healthcare professionals) Disconnection can seep into every aspect of the workplace, relationships especially. When we are separated from each other, and indeed ourselves, our human relationships are dumbed down into perfunctory superficiality, battles of egos and the compulsion for instant gratification. The potential power of service is subsumed in the actual struggles for personal power. The relationships at work mirror the nature of the corporate body. Disconnected organisations produce a disconnected workforce. Disconnected people produce disconnected organisations.

In such a culture, there is little room for the 'softer' things that seem to matter to people. Yet dis-spirited organisations carry hidden costs – high levels of attrition, sickness and burnout in the disconnected and dis-eased workforce that take their hidden toll on efficiency and productivity in the long term. The World Health Organization (1994) and the Health Education Authority (1996) both see burnout (the loss of function associated with stress), as a major cause of problems at work. Inadequate resources, lack of involvement in the decision-making process, excessive workloads and poor relationships in the workplace are all key factors. The impact on employees is higher levels of depression, hopelessness, despair, poor concentration and decision making, absenteeism, conflicts at home, physical illnesses, addiction to drugs and alcohol, and suicide.

If work organisations were just trench warfare, with plenty of recruits to fill the gaps left by those who fall, maybe it wouldn't matter too much as far as profitability or achieving targets were concerned. Yet leaving aside the grinding and insidious costs to an organisation of a less-than-happy workforce, there are the obvious costs of replacing and retraining people. One Confederation of British Industry (1999) survey put the costs to British industry of sickness due to stress as £5 billion. In the cutthroat world of business, is cutting the throats of the staff really the only way to succeed?

DISPIRITING WORDS

A couple of years ago the Royal College of Nursing conducted an extensive survey of the views of its members on the future of nursing (Wright et al., 1998), and the full report, available in RCN libraries, made some interesting points about nurses and their sense of alienation in the workplace. Pippa Gough, Brenda Poulton and I carried out the study and conducted a series of focus group exercises embracing over 2000 RCN members. A common thread was the sense of alienation from the workplace, which many nurses were, and still are, experiencing.

If spirituality means anything, it is about a sense of connection – with ourselves, each other, work and home and that which is beyond the self – whatever we perceive it to be. Dispirited workplaces create a sense of separation and disconnection; we become divorced from the satisfaction of a job well done and of a sense of right relationship with those we seek to serve – be they patients, clients or customers – and our colleagues. Organisations like this, dis-spirited, are far more likely to have higher levels of sickness and absenteeism and, in the case of health care, more patient dissatisfaction and greater risks of patient abuse.

Many factors can contribute to this sense of disconnection, and one of them is the signal given to staff through the language that is dominant in the organisation. The RCN study showed how nurses particularly loathed much of the terminology that pervades modern health care. Since the time of the study, I have shared its findings with many groups of different health professionals and it seems that nurses are not alone in their dislike. All kinds of therapists, doctors and other health-service workers feel alienated by the language used to govern the work they do.

> Reports, meetings, conferences, it was suggested, speak of 'key people' (but is not 'every member of staff a key person'?) or use the language of the business world ('take forward', 'downsizing', 'cost-effectiveness', 'value for money', 'evidence-based practice',

> *'benchmarking', 'business plans' . . . these and many others emerged as pet hates of*
> *respondents.*   Wright et al., 1998

Briskin (1998) illustrates how the business world seems to be increasingly addressing the significance of spirituality in the workplace – a message that has yet to get through to our healthcare system. And this includes a greater wariness of the language used and what message it conveys to its staff by its choice of words. The RCN study mentioned one particular bugbear – that of 'Human Resources'. When we have departments and staff with these words in their titles, what signals are we giving to colleagues about how they are valued (or not) by their employers? Resources are things we use, exploit. 'Human Resources' is a contradiction in terms, an industrial oxymoron – to be 'human' and to be a 'resource' suggest a jarring incompatibility. What is intended by the words is irrelevant – the perception of the receiver is all – if I am human how can you also see me as a resource, for by referring to me as the latter does not this at some level indicate a denial of my humanity?

'Human Resources' betrays a subconscious, and sometimes not so subconscious, element of the culture of health care and other organisations and how staff are seen. We have only to look at the state of the planet if we want to see the results of the mindset, which sees everything as a resource. We can transform health care by seriously re-thinking the workplace culture and what spirited relationships are all about. An indication that our health services are serious about a caring culture for staff would be the dumping of Human Resources terminology. I suspect workers in many different types of organisations experience the same sense of alienation when departments once dedicated to personnel or staff support are labelled, and indeed may function, to suggest that they are set up to get the most out of staff and control them, rather than nurture and encourage them. And please look at that word 'encourage' – derived from French roots (cœur = heart), it means to literally to fill with or give heart to something. Some of the language we use can make people feel they work in places that are soulless and heartless.

IS SOUL ANY BUSINESS OF BUSINESS?

There is compelling evidence, as suggested above, that the need for spiritual fulfilment is an integral part of being human. But is this something that should be left to the individual in their private time or is there a place for business, or any employing organisation for that matter, to take more of an interest, indeed action? Zohar and Marshall (2000) say that individuals and organisations that possess 'spiritual intelligence', that is to say actively seek, encourage and achieve meaning, purpose, connection, involvement and wholeness in all aspects of their being, are more likely to be happy, healthy and successful. Most employing organisations in commercially developed countries are bound by law to take care of their staff physically, mentally, socially and economically. But if spirituality is part of what it is to be human as well, just like our physiology and psychology, then it seems rational to presume that employers have a duty to support their staff in this dimension as well. Are we far off legislation compelling employers to meet certain spiritual needs of staff just as in many places they are compelled to provide minimum wages or pensions? Is the day close when employers will be sued by unhappy employees who became depressed because of the aggravation of a sense of disconnectedness at work through not being involved in decisions about their working lives? Are we close to trade unions pressing employers to set up quiet sanctuaries in the workplace for meditation, prayer and reflection?

Some organisations have recognised that treating staff well is part of a healthy, efficient and effective business, but the message does not yet seem to have got through to the majority. Even the NHS, Britain's largest employer (which you might think would, above all others, have the health of its workforce at the leading edge of its policies and practices) is still sadly lacking in this respect (Williams et al., 1998). Despite policy-making to improve support to staff in the workplace, such as the recent 'Working Lives' initiative, intended to produce more worker-friendly workplaces, reports of low morale and high attrition rates in the health services continue unabated. Even if the moral message of treating people humanely were difficult to take on board, you would think that the financial message would make more sit up and take notice. There is growing evidence that those who attend to the spiritual dimension of the workplace are more likely to be successful in what they do and be great places in which to work. Nourishing right relationships (Wright & Sayre-Adams, 2000) at work, which are based on shared decision making, trust, mutual support and a sense of meaning and purpose, all form part of a spiritual approach to the work ethic.

Is making money or being directed towards organisational targets compatible with caring and the spiritual support of staff in the workplace? One enterprising, internationally renowned doctor and writer on business ethics believes not. Deepak Chopra (1996) comments that 'when you focus on values, the economic side of life takes care of itself'. In other words, get the relationships right at work and whatever the organisation is set up to do it will do with a naturally following grace. Paying attention to getting all the goals and structures and systems right is putting the cart before the horse. Relationality first, *then* the system works. At the moment, huge amounts of energy are expended on getting the system right and then it is assumed the organisation will do what it's supposed to do. The reality stands in direct opposition to this. Goleman's thesis (1995) showed that organisations with what he called 'emotional intelligence', i.e. a sense of shared meaning, purpose, values and positive relationships at work, were far more likely to succeed. Likewise a Gallup report (Hatfield, 1999) found the most profitable and/or successful organisations were more likely to be those that actively promoted spiritual values and practices in the workplace. Thus a picture begins to emerge that enterprising and energetic companies and other organisations are likely to succeed in their goals when their foundations pay attention to soul first and systems second. Such entities are likely to be even more successful when they adopt approaches that nourish the spirits as well as the salaries of their staff.

This means a lot more than investing in a crèche, better pay scales and access to aerobics or massage for the workers. Yet it doesn't have to cost a lot and the methods available are tried and tested throughout history, providing mentoring, support and spiritual counselling in the workplace; developing practices that support personal spiritual awareness, such as meditation and building communities and ways of conducting ourselves at work that generate a sense of support and connection. Add to these – team-building exercises, time out together, access to rest and recuperation facilities, time for reflection and other techniques that deepen personal insights, motivation and the positive aspects of working relationships with colleagues and the organisation as a whole, and that which lies beyond the organisation. All of these and more, directed to encouraging a sense of meaning and purpose in the workplace and focused on what right relationships, truth and highest values mean to people, show how the goals of the organisation can be wedded to success without sacrificing kindness and compassion, welfare for other human beings and indeed all of creation. Matthew Fox (1994) believes that the task that lies ahead of us is enormous, because he calls for nothing less than a complete re-enchantment of the workplace and a re consecration of work. A sceptic may balk at these words. Can the drudgery of work that so many know day in and day out ever be seen and felt as holy? It is easy to see this might be so for people like myself who have the privilege of doing work that is fulfilling. My work allows me considerable personal control and into it I can weave my spiritual life so that any sense of being spiritual in some things and not in others simply disappears. How much more difficult must it be for the woman on the production line or the child in the sweatshop or the man down the pit?

As Briskin (1998) points out, work that offers a deep sense of spirituality – purpose, meaning, fulfilment, connected to 'all that is', serving God, however we experience it – currently seems to be a minority sport the way much of our economy and social structures are organised. In this context, Matthew Fox's urgings are revolutionary and will demand nothing less than a complete rethink in the way we organise human work activity. Meanwhile, an old saying holds true: 'Nobody ever died wishing they had spent more time at the office.'

Most workers in Britain, and perhaps worldwide, would understand how Sisyphus felt. Condemned by the gods, his task was to eternally roll a huge

boulder uphill. Labouring to the point of collapse, he would complete his struggle, only to see the boulder roll downhill again, for him once more to repeat his
labour. It doesn't have to be like this. We can be enterprising and efficient and
still work from an ethical and spiritual basis in harmony with the workforce,
society and the wider creation. There is hope for this, as many organisations that
are choosing to work ethically and spiritually are demonstrating. Lerner (2000)
leaves us with an optimistic message suggesting that the old way of working will
pass. The grand sweep of history tells us that nothing lasts for long.

> *It will pass because people hunger for a deeper kind of recognition from each other than
> the current organisation of society allows. It will change because people hunger for lives
> in which their spiritual needs are not just relegated to the sidelines and to their weekends,
> but rather fully expressed and integrated into our daily lives. It will change because people
> need to live in a world based on love and on caring for each other. It will change because
> people are coming to recognise the intrinsic connection between the ecological crisis and
> the values of individualism and selfishness enshrined in the competitive market. It will
> change because people need a world whose social institutions are based on a joint sense
> of awe and wonder at the universe and on a collective understanding of our role as
> stewards of and nurturers of Gaia. It will change because people will take their own
> understanding of the Unity of All Being seriously.*

My uncle was a farmer. Maybe he was luckier than most because he still
farmed in the way he wanted, had relationality in his work and never had to
work on a factory production line. He was a humble and simple man with simple tastes. He spent hours with me as a child walking over the land. He had no
grand ambitions, just to be in his home, work the land, love his wife. I think of
him sometimes and the part played by Marlon Brando in the film *On The Water-
front* when he wails in his despair, 'I could have been somebody, I could have
been a contender.' Some merchant came to the farm once and I listened thumb
in mouth and watched my uncle. The man promised investment, an expansion
of the farm, and ideas for new ways of working. He would make my uncle rich.
When he got rich, he would have more free time to enjoy life he told him.

My uncle never wanted to be a contender, and he was content in the somebody he was. When the merchant left, my uncle mumbling goodbyes and
promises to think about it, he and I walked to the front of the farmhouse. The
sun was setting and you could see the mayflies hanging in the air in the
summer heat. We leaned on the fence and watched the sun go down; my uncle
had a wry smile on his face. He spat out, 'Free time, eh?', then chuckled, 'This
costs nowt, lad'. And he waved his arm to the hills and the clouds and the swal-
lows passing over the meadow. We went inside for supper into the hot kitchen
with the smell of currant buns and tea. My uncle worked till he dropped, the
farm never got any bigger and he and my aunt never got any richer, and I never
heard him complain once.

CHAPTER 3
FAITH AND THE DONKEY STONE — THE DEATH OF CREDIBILITY

Some patients recover simply because of their satisfaction with the goodness of their doctor.

Hippocrates (Dalrymple, 2000)

A WORSHIP AT THE ALTAR OF CLEANLINESS

I grew up on a working class estate to the north of Manchester. It was the kind of place where everybody knew everybody else – and everybody else's business, or at least thought they did! The churches of various denominations, closely followed by the pubs, betting shops, working men's clubs and corner shops, formed the social glue that bound the community together. It was filled with its given rituals, its ways of doing things. Outcasts they were who did not conform. I remember Mrs Peacock, an 'old woman' who refused to 'act her age' but wore make-up and 'dressed to the nines'; or the Mason family who rocked the street with the scandal of divorce; or Michael, the lonely boy who was ostracised because his mother had 'gone mental'. It was a community which did not travel much, either to foreign parts (and 'foreign' would have been the next town, let alone another country) or up or down the social scale, or in the realms of the imagination.

This was, after all, post-war England and the country was only slowly dragging itself out of the glory of victory on the battlefield but the penury of a lost economy. All those grainy black and white pictures I saw a little later in life – *A Taste of Honey* or *Room at the Top* or *Saturday Night and Sunday Morning* – my home, upbringing and social mores were just like these. Except, looking back, it does not have so much the quality of a film as a still photograph. A time held fixed by its own certainties that were soon to slip away, changed forever, but not necessarily for the better, to paraphrase Lennon and McCartney in the song 'In My Life'.

People then believed in certain things, or at least gave the impression that they did. They believed in respect for 'elders and betters' – the doctor, the teacher, the nurse, the factory owner, the landlord, the vicar. The slow decline in church attendance had yet to make its mark. Church was still a focus for community activity – the youth club, Sunday school, the festival events. Grandest of all of the last of these were the 'Whit Walks' – the Whitsuntide massed parades in the streets when whole towns would dress in their finest and line the streets to see thousands of people marching behind brass bands and banners. Every church, Sunday school group, and girl guide or boy scout troupe would put on its finest for all the world to see. They would march in long columns for what seemed like endless miles – tough little boys made to behave for a day, uncomfortable in smart shirts and ties, eager to be out of them and join in the after-Walks games. The girls more sedate in fine dresses, the product of months of labour and penny pinching and the subject of proud smiles and uttered 'oohs' and 'aaahs'.

Within a generation all this was gone. My mother hung on to her values and way of doing things to the last. Until she died, she continued to do the same things the women had always done. Scrimp and save. Raise children. Feed the husband. And clean. Some people believed in God. My mother, she believed in cleaning.

The house was always spotless. She seemed to have spent her life on her knees in her own ritual prayer to the god of household hygiene. And, regular as clockwork she would, like all but a few of the women in the street, clean the doorstep. This was above all others to me the most bizarre and incomprehensible of rituals. Not only was the front doorstep washed and scrubbed, it was then religiously rubbed with the 'donkey stone' – a hand-sized square block of stone, creamy coloured. Elbows and hands would ache in the labour over each step. Left to dry, it transformed a dull, grey concrete step into a honey-coloured slab at the entrance to each door. It was a sign to all with eyes to see and brains to comprehend that this house was a clean house, a respectable house. A house without was a house of shame, of lower moral standards, of people who were not as good as us.

Anyone reading this who does not hail from an English working-class background could be forgiven a degree of incredulity. Yet, the donkey stone ritual had no purpose other than a symbolic one. It was not antiseptic. It was of doubtful aesthetics. But it told you a lot about the people who lived in that house, and more importantly, the woman of that house. People believed in donkey stones. It is the nature of such beliefs, such small insignificant practices, that in accumulation are the stuff that binds a people together. It was part of the way things were; the agreed shared order of a community, the central core of the common ground that holds all else together.

THE TIDE OF DISBELIEF

It's worth remembering a line from the Yeat's poem cited in Chapter 1, how things fall apart when the centre does not hold. This slipping away of cultural norms happens when we lose faith in ways of thinking about and doing things. Things fall apart when we no longer believe in them. No system – religious, political or social – seems able to stand against the tide of disbelief. It has happened in my lifetime to the culture that birthed and nourished me, and is now long gone. It has happened in the swift collapse of communism in Eastern Europe. It is happening now in the explosion of Internet information that is eroding the power base of those who once held knowledge and services exclusively. It is happening, too, in an enormous shift of values, as Paul Ray's (1996) and the 'I-Society' (Thomas, 1999) studies have illustrated. Religion, conformity, authority are 'out'; personal growth, deepening self-awareness, the spiritual search are 'in' for an ever-growing part of the population in the West.

Prigogine and Stenders (1984) see this collapse of shared values as 'dissipation' – a loss of energy and drive from a given way of being. This is not a complete loss, however, or a decline into nothingness or chaos. Rather, the phenomenon is not so much the death of a system as a reconfiguration, a natural process that occurs in all belief systems from time to time, driven by many factors, which produces the emergence of a new order.

Just as Ireland, Australia and the USA have recently witnessed a fall from grace and power of the Catholic Church, fuelled by numerous scandals around the behaviour of its priests and nuns, so a similar pattern has emerged affecting healthcare professionals. Many public surveys show how enormously popular people like doctors and nurses still are. What has steadily dissipated is the once near-absolute faith in them that the men and women like my parents once held. Media reports of failing professionals have accelerated the demolition job on the bastions of professional power. In the UK, the serial killers nurse Beverly Allitt and doctor Harold Shipman (whose cases have arisen against a background of endless press reports of botched operations, faulty test results, failed heart surgery on children and the absence of informed consent to many procedures) have added their influence to the momentum.

It matters little that most practitioners may be sound in their work. What is dying is not so much the popularity of these professions, rather their credibility. They find their authority being questioned and tested as never before. As Dalrymple (2000) has recently pointed out, 'If we trust our doctor, we trust his treatment; and if we trust his treatment, it is more likely to cure us.' The same can be said of all the professionals from nurse to hospital chaplain, social worker to teacher. Faith, belief and trust in the professional are an integral part of the effectiveness of treatment and care. Things fall apart when this centre does not hold. When the professional cannot be seen to be trustworthy, what is at stake is more than an undermining of their professional power and authority. More than their livelihoods are at risk. People's health is at risk too. The potential of the emotional trigger towards healing (Pert, 1997) is diminished. In search of health and healing, people will naturally turn elsewhere; not only toward treatments they can trust, but also towards practitioners they can trust too.

EROSION OF THE SYSTEM

We can lose faith in both people and systems, and the NHS, often held up as one of the world's great pioneering humanitarian examples, is suffering like the professions from the same loss of faith. Whether the government of the day as I write, with its promises of more investment, will restore that faith remains to be seen. Let me give you a couple of recent examples. I could tell you of my sister, crippled by pain from a failing hip, who could wait no longer and eventually 'went private'. Of a friend in deep distress, but whose surgeon 'did not believe in' the complementary therapies, so saw no role for them in supporting her at a time of crisis. Of a dear woman with breast cancer whose admission was delayed because of bed shortages. All these people, the tip of the iceberg I believe, are not the mobile middle classes. They are solid working class folks who have 'paid their stamp' for decades. Yet they opted out. The NHS was limiting access to choices and promptness of treatment. No doubt their choices saved the NHS money, but they, like thousands of others, no longer have faith in the NHS. It was not there for them when and in the way they needed it.

It also occurs to me that it may not be long before the science catches up with the lawyers – the field of psychoneuroimmunology, for example, where the link between stress and ill health is being demonstrated (Pert, 1997). Will my friend with breast cancer seek compensation because the stress of delayed admission exacerbated her condition? Will my neighbour with the post-op wound infection seek some redress because the lack of psychological support increased her fear, suppressing her immune response and thus worsening her suffering? I can see the claim files piling up on the desks of our healthcare administrators right now.

Meanwhile, those opposed to a state-funded system have spotted the opportunity this loss of faith presents. Seeing the crack in the belief in the system, they have found the place to drive the wedge of discontent. Accelerating the loss of faith in the NHS, they can move the agenda on to the search for 'better' alternatives. The fall of the NHS will therefore not be due to lack of nurses, or longer waiting lists or limited choices, but the effect that factors like these have on people. Remember Eastern Europe. No matter how powerful and permanent the systems seemed to be, in the end they fell apart when enough people no longer believed in them.

Perhaps money will have stemmed the tide and restored faith in the NHS by the time this book has gone to press. My own belief in the NHS is still there, but I see all around me examples of the steady erosion of faith in it. I am a child of the NHS, a product of the post-second World War reforming Labour government. Levels of state-funded health, social and educational care had been introduced, which meant that I had help and opportunities undreamed of by my parents. I grew up more secure, better educated and healthier than was possible for working-class people a generation before. And in the case of health care in particular, it had become fear-less; not in the sense that sickness and what it might mean were any less threatening, but a primary fear of not being able to pay for proper health care had been removed.

Maybe tackling some of the root disgruntlements with the modern system with more funds will work, but without a wholesale restoration of belief in the NHS and those professionals who serve it, this form of spiritual crisis will follow its inexorable course. The crisis is indeed spiritual because it is all about faith, meaning, purpose and connection. And a spiritual crisis needs spiritual solutions.

It will take a good deal more than some tinkering with the system, such as changing the regulatory mechanisms governing healthcare practitioners or pumping money into a creaky system. Trust in professionals and systems like the NHS (and most healthcare practitioners still work in the NHS; the privately funded approaches remain the choice of a minority) is only partially founded on notions of public accountability. It will take a wholesale reappraisal and re-enactment of public−professional relationships, and a new paradigm that is grounded in partnerships, dialogue and honesty. The search for that quality of relationship by patients with professionals is evident in the turning towards complementary therapies and therapists − right relationship as well as an effective helper is what people in need are seeking.

THE COMPLEMENTARY APPROACH

The longest word in the English language has only two letters and I heard it recently as I sat in the reception area at the Bristol Cancer Help Centre. A woman arrived looking tense, pale and exhausted, leaned on the reception desk and looked around her, then just moved off to one side and sat beside me, sinking into the armchair. She let out a long 'Aaaah' − so long in fact that it would take a full line or two of 'a's to capture the full length of it. With a sound of only two letters, she spoke volumes.

The centre in Bristol has been a world leader in offering an holistic approach to cancer care, and part of the story has been the successful integration of the complementary therapies. After years of scepticism, indeed outright hostility, the approaches it pioneered are now increasingly part of mainstream health care. More research is being dedicated to evaluating the effects of complementary and alternative medicine (CAM), as a recent report (Duffin, 2003) has outlined. The demand to know 'what works' using standard scientific criteria (e.g. randomised double-blind controlled trials) seems reasonable, but these therapies do not lend themselves easily to such scrutiny. Relying as most trials do upon detectable physiological impacts of, say, the application of a substance such as an aromatherapy oil, seems hopelessly wide of the mark in seeking to get at how CAM works. There are too many subtle factors at play, just as there are, it may be argued, with orthodox medicine, where much evidence suggests that outcomes are as much affected by the relationships with the healthcare practitioner, the context of care and so on as the physiological impact of a drug.

Often dismissed as the 'placebo effect' by the scientific establishment, we are talking here about the uncanny ability of human beings to get better even when they have been given a 'neutral' substance (Peters, 2002). The capacity of some scientists to dismiss an effect simply because it cannot be (easily) explained takes the breath away. It seems peculiar that the ability for a human being to experience some form of healing when *not* given a treatment (but believing they have been) has often been dismissed as mind over matter. Leaving aside the issue that science really struggles to explain 'mind', or considering how cheap medicine could be if we just gave out low-cost placebo drugs, something profound has been largely ignored – how we feel and believe something is happening actually makes something happen.

It is estimated that in the UK 15–20 million people have consulted a CAM practitioner at some point in their lives and that currently 5 million people do so each year (Foundation for Integrated Medicine, 2003), spending some £1.6 billion – and so the demands are increasing to make CAM more available on the NHS and to demonstrate 'what works'. Like faith in the professionals and health delivery systems, faith in treatments is equally significant. Credibility – belief that a treatment being used will help, when delivered in a system we believe in and in a relationship with professionals where we trust and believe in them with equal strength – is a mightily potent force for health and wellbeing. Many orthodox professionals have invested a lot of time and effort into rubbishing the complementary therapies and those who practise and make use of them. But there is no doubting the tide of public opinion moving towards CAM. While there are signs of change, with increasing numbers of orthodox practitioners willing to embrace and integrate CAM approaches, the divisions still run deep.

What places like the Bristol Centre are doing is showing how an integrated approach can work. And it is not just integration of treatments, but also paying attention to people's belief systems – in their treatments, their carers, the system they are using. These too, as much as any drug or surgery, are part of the healing and curing process.

A PLACE FOR MYTH AND RITUAL?

As a student nurse I fell for the lot. I happily went to theatre for a long stand, to the supplies department for a set of fallopian tubes and set up a bed for a fractured tonsil at night sister's request. Not to mention the clingfilm over the loo trick. I won't argue with those who might call me exceptionally stupid or naïve, but 30 years ago you just did what your elders and betters told you – and joined in the hysterics afterwards.

I wonder if the healthcare students of today experience such humorous rites of passage towards professionalism? Such rituals were not just practical jokes – they had meaning and purpose. They affirmed the social hierarchy and provided humour as a means of releasing stress in a difficult work world.

Rituals in nursing and other parts of health care have had something of a bad press in recent years, in the push for evidence-based practice and rationalistic health care. Walsh and Ford (1989) and Ford and Walsh (1994) produced particularly strong arguments for questioning myth and ritual in nursing. While some practices may have been unhelpful and downright dangerous (like applying Mercurochrome to pressure sores), this does not mean that all ritual practices are dismissible simply because they are just that – ritual. Some have suggested that rituals are in fact profoundly important in bonding groups of workers together, as a means of dealing with stress and providing certainty and common purpose (Biley & Wright, 1997; Holland, 1993). Once again, this time in the case of healthcare workers, we come across the significance of believing in something, even if it does not at first glance have any rational basis to it.

It is interesting, for example, that stress and burnout rates among nurses and other carers have risen coincidentally with this change of culture – an increasing emphasis on efficiency and effectiveness in the workplace, the passing of uniforms and hats, the loss of communal breaks on shift systems without overlaps and minimalist staffing levels. There may be a side effect of these changes, which we have overlooked.

Please don't get me wrong, I'm not arguing for a return to harmful practices. But I do suggest that not all myth and ritual is wrong, for it provides a hugely potent means of providing mutual support and collective action and purpose – ask any religious organisation! If our old rituals have passed away, what does seem to be important is that we forge new ones to replace them as a key means of support to both staff and patients. What can we do to build effective teams if working patterns inhibit opportunities for staff to get together

(Lee, 2001)? What approaches to 'saying goodbye' can we adopt in a secular age if 'last offices' (see Chapter 21) is reduced to wrapping a body and removing it from the ward as quickly as possible?

Hammer et al. (1992) have illustrated the work of nurses who put a white cloth on a table with dim candlelight upon it. They sang songs and read the names of the dead children out loud. All this to help them release their feelings of sadness and loss and to restore their capacity to continue looking after terminally ill children. Schroeder-Sheker (1994) has done groundbreaking work in the newly emerging field of music thanatology – staff and patients composing and using music as ritual accompaniment for the dying.

Finding the right place for new myths and rituals in health care (and perhaps restoring some old ones) may not be contrary to modern evidence-based practice. The return of the matron, for example, to the NHS is more than a political gimmick or an unnecessary backward step, as some in the media have argued. The whole point of myths and rituals is that they are not grounded in obvious reason and scientific evidence – they are used because they work for people, because they have meaning and significance to us. Regardless of what matrons do or do not do, the symbolic significance of their presence to patients, and perhaps to staff, is something that we cannot overlook. Myths, symbols and rituals matter to people. A scientific analysis of a Beethoven symphony could provide us with every detail of the notes used, the structure of the harmonics, the placing of every instrument – but it can never illuminate for us what it means to us or how we feel and behave when we hear it.

CHRISTMAS? HUMBUG!

I was musing on myth and ritual during a cold winter's day in Sheffield. The city seemed to undergo a shopping enema. It was late afternoon in December and some sort of collective evacuation was under way as masses of people armed with bags of Christmas goodies piled on to trams and buses. I'd arrived for a conference and thought to head for the cathedral for evensong, a restorative moment after a busy week with more to come. The great gates were locked, the cathedral closed at 4 p.m. Against the flow of shoppers I decided to walk around the grand building in the fading light, and found only sealed doors and not a glimmer of light from within. At the rear, by the steps of the east window, a glassy eyed man was shooting up, oblivious to my presence.

This little scene touched me as a metaphor for the loss of meaning in Christmas, or more precisely, a shift of meaning from something that was of profound significance to something somehow more base and shallow – the dumbing down of Christ's Mass into a vast, collective pig-out on food and drink and gifts. Recent estimates suggest that each of us will spend about £600 this Christmas on this orgy of giving and receiving. Pre-Christian pagans or heathens (both words being used pejoratively in our culture, yet originally referring to people 'of the country/heath' – immersed in the divinity of nature and the creation and without a formal religious creed) are often dismissed as being godless. Yet their festivals were one of worship and reverence for the gods and goddesses as they saw them. Early Christians had to adapt to these festivals, and so Christmas emerged at the winter solstice – bringing new meaning to that symbolic time of the longest night, which also signalled the lengthening days to come. The return of the light to the world became linked to the birth of Jesus; the new and consummate symbol of the divine light upon the earth (even though all the scholarly, theological evidence actually points to Jesus being born much earlier in the year, perhaps in spring or early autumn).

The modern spirit of Christmas has, for huge numbers of people, lost its theistic spiritual significance and become instead a material sacrifice on a monumental scale. The shopping malls have become the new temples; the giving of gifts with their hints of value equated with love, the new rituals; the TV ads the new chants and dogmas. It's not even Pagan, for this new religion that is capturing the world is utterly godless. And the price of that is the emptiness that lies at the heart of this ersatz merry-mass. The food and alcohol and the glittering pressies, and the fat jolly snowmen, twinkly trees and Santas (and there's another irony – the Santa creation and the Christmas tree have Pagan, Shamanic roots) bear witness to a culture that has become materially wealthy but spiritually poor. The escalating suicide and depression rates at this time, the crimes of violence and theft, the family wars when the attempts at sherry-drowned bonhomie collapse under the weight of their own repressed fury – these and others bear witness to the fundamental disconnectedness that lies beneath. The manic desire to spend, eat or drink more is like an insatiable addiction – filling the emptiness of the god-shaped hole in our consciousness with anything, especially if it is readily purchasable and consumable, to keep away the existential angst.

When we seek to find meaning in material ephemera, then we must face the loss of that meaning when the fun of the gifts is past, when the hysteria of the party is awakened in the cold light of day when the booze wears off. For some people this is OK, and perhaps it was for me once. Maybe I'm just turning into a grumpy old man, but on reflection the hollowness of the Christmas binge was never enough for me. And I think I am not alone in finding the loss of connection, meaning and purpose fundamentally dissatisfying in the annual spendfest.

My family and friends made some conscious shifts a few years ago to reduce the materialism of Christmas. We cut back on the mass tree demolition known as posting the Christmas cards and gave the money to charity instead. We gave gifts, but limited the cost to £10 or, preferably, something you had made yourself. And the party set to celebrate the season is a gathering of song and dance drawn from sacred traditions. These little ways of downshifting are not about being a party pooper, although I'm sure not a few readers would see it in that light. Nor are we being prohibitionist – there is food and wine aplenty. It's just that we have for many years now found that sometimes less is more. Christmas time becomes a more enjoyable family and friendly occasion when we remind ourselves of what it's really all about and tune into its essential and authentic spirit: a time to reaffirm the light of love in our lives whether you are a Christian or not, but specifically to celebrate the birth of this hugely special being if you are. Holding a sense of reverence and the sacred at special times does not have to be a killjoy affair; in fact it can be quite the reverse.

I recall the profound effects on patients of the midnight carol-singing procession through the wards by lamplight – with nurses and doctors looking the part. I remember being the charge nurse and arriving early to make bacon butties for staff and patients, and then carving the turkey at dinner. My children came to the ward with me on Christmas day and, oh, what fun they had giving the presents to patients with Father Christmas, and going round the ward with the vicar, and helping to serve drinks. And, yes, how they enjoyed it, but no – nowhere near as much as the patients, radiant in their appreciation of these precious gifts – of time, attention, sincere wellwishing – low in materials, high in love.

In the industrial process that has become much of modern health care, so many little gestures like these have now been lost. Some staff still put in the effort; it's not all lost although it's against the grain of 'efficiency'. But, heck, they meant something – and meaning and purpose and connection are what spirituality and Christmas are all about. They make us feel better, and people who feel better are more likely to get better.

In the cold shadows of the cathedral I watched the man and his drugs and the glazed look in his eyes. I watched the eyes of shoppers piling on to the bus. And they looked the same.

The professionals involved in health care, wherever and whoever they may be, are going to have to come to terms with credicide – the death of belief in general and in themselves specifically. Paul Hodgkin has noted (1996) the:

> ... death of belief. Not this or that one but all and every. Strictly speaking of course it means the active killing of belief rather than just its simple demise. Some dark agent has been out mugging belief in the night, jumping it, slicing it up while our eyes were turned to see what the arc lights of the media were bringing us this time.

It may not be possible to recreate what has been, but it may be possible for those of us involved in health care to gather the dissipation and reconfigure it into newly forged relationships and practices for health and healing. To rebuild a centre which holds, for a while at least. For some, healing relationships of this sort will be nothing new. Many practitioners have learned the arts of right relationship with patients and clients. For others, however, hooked into the old authoritarian way of being with people or obsessed by the rational-scientific paradigm, it will demand nothing less than wholesale transformation. In the respiriting of health, we who are healthcare practitioners can participate in this change or become the donkey stones of our time.

The Bristol Cancer Help Centre tel: 0845 123 2310, www.bristolcancerhelp.org

CHAPTER 4
THANK GOD FOR BURNOUT

Suffering is part of our training programme for becoming wise.

Ram Dass, 2002

THE BURNED-OUT HEALTHCARE WORKER – A SPIRITUAL CRISIS

Anyone who has experienced burnout will tell you it's a tough place to be – very tough. Your whole life seems to collapse around you. Normal conversations can become a monumental effort. Relationships crack and break under the strain. Everyday activities are transformed so that even the simplest of tasks becomes an exhausting labour. The work you once looked forward to fills you with dread. Physical ailments of all kinds assail you, emotions bounce between extremes, minor irritations become monumental problems. Meaning, purpose and joy in work and life are crushed by hopelessness and despair. Nothing seems right any more. We literally lose faith – in work, in life, in relationships, in ourselves.

A dispirited healthcare environment (see Chapters 1 and 2) is contributing significantly to the high levels of stress and burnout that healthcare practitioners experience, often in higher numbers than comparable occupations (Wright & Sayre-Adams, 2000). My experience at the Sacred Space Foundation (a UK charity with retreat and recuperation facilities for those in burnout; see contact details at the end of this chapter), where we help over 400 people a year, leads me to believe that if there is a difference with other occupational groups it's a narrow one. Teachers, executives, social workers, chaplains, builders – you name it, the chances are that somebody from that line of work has been here seeking escape from and resolution of their suffering.

Seeing burnout as an opportunity can be a tall order if you are stuck in it. It's scary; the current landscape seems barren, the journey beyond it is full of unknowns and there is no sight of a possible distant shore where things might be better. Many try to drown the pain with drugs or drink or serial relationships or whatever it takes to shut out the awesome darkness that is creeping up on them. Others hang on in there, waiting for something better to come along or for the next holiday. Unfortunately, the grass may be greener on the other side of the hill; it's just that there's another hill there as well. And as to the holiday – we take a break from the workplace in some foreign clime and have temporary respite from the ongoing struggle. Unfortunately after only a few hours back at work we can feel things are just like they always were. Nothing has changed.

HOLIDAYS AND HOLY-DAYS

Holidays are helpful: they can give us the breather we need from ordinary reality to re-collect and re-energise ourselves. But, people in burnout need more. Indeed the original meaning of the word 'holiday' is a holy day – a time not only to take a break from work because of a religious commemoration, but also a time to become more holy (whole). Whole and holy have the same linguistic roots – the Teutonic *hal* or *hael* or *hail* meaning hale, whole, hearty. Further back in Middle-Eastern languages we find them related to concepts of oneness, all, the holy one. Indeed, someone in burnout will often say that they need to 'get myself together' – reflecting that sense of disorientation, disconnection and fragmentation that comes with it. What those with burnout need, therefore, are true (w)holy-days – time to explore their experience, find ways through and beyond it and emerge into a new and healthy whole. This type of (w)holy-day enables an integration, a transformation, of who and what we are in the world. After a holiday we go back to work pretty much as we left it. After a (w)holy-day we may go back to work, but at another level we do not go back. Some change or shift has occurred within us, some expansion of consciousness and greater awareness of who we are has taken place in us. So, while we go back to work in body with little observable change as far as the outside world is concerned, within ourselves we are never quite the same again, and deal with work in quite different ways so that we never get into that burnout abyss again if we stay awake and true to ourselves.

The challenge of burnout is to treat it for what it is – a spiritual crisis. Work pressures have lots to do with it, it's true, but these are often the *agents provocateurs* rather than the root causes. Burnout is the desperate cry of the soul to break free. It is the time of the collapse of the ego, when the soul refuses to live any longer as it has and is punching through to get home. A spiritual crisis is a crisis of meaning, purpose and connection, and so is burnout. Everything that we once thought of as normal or valuable or certain in our lives can suddenly be thrown into turmoil. Psychotherapist and author Frances Vaughan (1995) writes that:

> *Anyone who has experienced burnout, a common occupational hazard among helping professionals, has probably had the feeling of being trapped in a web of necessity and impossible demands. Most recommended treatments for burnout consist of stress reduction or setting boundaries. They overlook the fact that burnout usually indicates a state of spiritual aridity, and the effective treatment may call for spiritual renewal or awakening the soul.*

A spiritual crisis demands spiritual solutions – no amount of juggling work-loads or changing jobs or setting boundaries will challenge the fundamental assault upon the ego that burnout represents. This is not a time to take a holi-day but a (w)holy-day – a time to feel more 'whole' and to allow our deepest needs for meaning and purpose in life to surface and find true expression once again in our work. By permitting this long 'aha' moment, we are enabled to see through the illusions by which we have been living, and come to rest in a new way of being in the world – a way that no longer wounds us, and at the same time makes us infinitely more able to be of service to others without burning ourselves out.

BURNOUT AS A BLESSING

A successful passage through burnout can make such a shift in our way of being in the world that we will wonder why on earth we did not see this before. It may also lead us to see, perhaps with gratitude, what a blessing the suffering of burnout was. Had it not happened, we would still be struggling as before. It can literally be a born-again feeling as we come to feel so much more connected to all that is, to see through illusions and experience a deeper reality and per-haps our God, whoever or whatever we perceive that to be. The suffering of burnout is real and visceral, but with the right sort of support and guidance, it can be a journey from one shore to another, lovingly and safely, that brings us to a new landscape of spiritual wellbeing.

Someone wrote to me recently in a state of deep unhappiness and despera-tion. She described all the classic symptoms of burnout, but felt utterly alone, like she was the only one who was experiencing this problem. She felt worse because she had a problem – everything about herself told her that she should be able to cope, that there was something wrong or unworthy about herself because she could not. This is another aspect of burnout – the 'double wham-my' – not only do the symptoms make us feel so awful, but we beat ourselves up with guilt and shame. She knew she had burnout, but was further afraid that her general practitioner would want her to see a counsellor and a psychiatrist, and to start antidepressants.

She was right in her self-diagnosis. Burnout rarely comes like a thunderbolt but steals up on you over the years like a fog creeping slowly into your life – then one day you wake up and realise you just can't see your way through it.

She was right also in her letter to observe that the stress of the job was only part of the cause. People can try and trick their way out of burnout by changing jobs. A temporary respite may follow but sure enough the fog finds a way back in again. I say this not to remove the responsibility of employers to provide nurturing environments for the staff; however, it is important to examine (and this can be a tough one) what processes are at work in ourselves that draw us to and keep us in such a wounding situation. Burnout is not purposeless – it is a sign that we can no longer tolerate aspects of our working life that no longer have heart and meaning for us. Our psyche is collapsing under the weight of things that it simply cannot hack anymore.

There is hope, however; for just as burnout is a sign that something in us is dying, it is also signifying that something is waiting to be born. Burnout is not a disease but a symptom, and by paying attention to what is really going on inside us we can pass beyond it. Who knows what lies beyond? Our hearts know. I recall a dentist recently who came to realise after 20 years that he no longer wanted to be a dentist but to work with computers; a policeman who really was ready to leave and study horticulture; a doctor at the peak of her profession who wanted to be a full-time mother; a physiotherapist who longed to break free and teach horse riding. Burnout is an inner voice telling us to move into what does have heart and meaning for us – it may be demanding a change in work or relationships, or changing the way we are, in existing work and relationships. For some it embraces a wholesale reappraisal of their lives and their values, and leads them into the deep soul work of seeking to connect more meaningfully with their God, however that is manifested for them (the 'whosoever, whatsoever' as Rabbi Lionel Blue (2001) calls 'it'). For others it is surrendering to a new career path that is right for them, and overcoming all the obstacles to get there (Glouberman, 2002).

One of the ways out of burnout is to take charge of it and that can start by finding out more from the likes of others who have gone through it too. Those who are in the midst of it need to know that they are not alone and they are not crazy. It is difficulty to quantify the numbers experiencing burnout, as the subject seems to be lost under the general topic of the high levels of stress at work (see Chapter 2). I am certain, after 20 years' experience, that the numbers we are dealing with at the Foundation are but the tip of a very large iceberg. In a world where 'God is dead' (see Chapter 1) I also suspect that a contributing factor is that without the foundation of something 'other' to turn to, a deeper Self, all we have is ourselves, and the transient self – our personhood, our ego – is a fragile basis for rock-solid strength in the world.

Counsellors and psychiatrists may be able to help, and it is interesting how many healthcare professionals are willing to dish out the pills to others but horrified at the thought that they may have to take antidepressants themselves. Even so, the drugs are OK in the short term, like a crutch if we break a leg, to get us through a crisis. They may be more problematic, indeed counterproductive, in the long term or may inhibit the deeper work that needs to be undertaken, by glossing over the present situation and providing a veneer of coping. The risk with conventional counselling or psychotherapy or psychiatry is that the person can get labelled with a diagnosis, a 'problem' that needs to be 'fixed'. Skilled helpers with burnout see it for what it is, an opportunity within the crisis. What the burned-out person needs is a special kind of counselling where someone will come alongside them, knowing what they are going through and, like the best of midwives, see the person not as sick but ready to give birth. This kind of spiritual midwifery, as Margaret Guenther (2002) calls it, sees the person not as a problem to be fixed, but a soul waiting to be birthed into the world through the womb of their current existence.

CHANGING THE WORLD – STAYING THE SAME

One of the features of burnout, at least in the early stages, is the tendency to fall into victim behaviour – 'This is happening to me because of my hostile boss/poor staff levels/my nasty partner/my unsupportive colleagues.' Such a view can keep us stuck and prevent us from facing up to what is really going on. That is not to say that there aren't inhospitable workplaces and relationships that need addressing. Rather it is also important to see these in the overall context of what is going on, especially if projecting all our woes onto them is keeping us from what might be the tougher work of dealing with what we might be bringing to the situation.

I am reminded of a ward sister I worked with in my early nursing days. She worked hard, harder than most. The ward was spotlessly clean and the patients with their shining faces lined up by their beds each morning were a suitable match. Sometimes the ward was busy, sometimes quiet, but this dedicated ward sister, I knew, never made such distinctions. No matter who asked the question, or when it was asked, 'How are things on the ward today?' always had the same response.

'It's awful', 'We're overworked', 'There's not enough staff' – mantra-like they spilled from her lips, though half the beds may be empty and the ward flooded with staff by a concerned nursing officer. Things could *never* get better in her eyes, no matter what efforts were made.

I used to think that she was a one-off or maybe the ward really was frantic and I, behind my plastic apron as I drifted from bed to bed, was missing something. Open the page of any nursing or other healthcare journal and you will find, among the (relatively rare) success stories, a vast collective whinge about our lot. No matter what governments or managers or leaders do to make life better for us, they are often greeted with the same old negativity and doubts. No matter what the policy or proposal, a huge part of the body politic of healthcare professionals (and none are exempt from it) responds with a collective wail of disapproval.

That is not to say there aren't serious flaws within our healthcare systems. Nursing, medicine and other therapies can be tough professions to work in and we often struggle with time and resources. But there may be a little more to the picture than the stereotypical overworked staff and the uncaring employer. Sogyal Rinpoche (1992) notes how:

> *Our contemporary education indoctrinates us in the glorification of doubt, has created in fact what could almost be called a religion or theology of doubt, in which to be seen to be intelligent we have to be seen to doubt everything, to always point to what's wrong and rarely to ask what's right or good, cynically to denigrate all inherited ideals and philosophies, or any theory that is done in simple goodwill or an innocent heart.*

Such a culture of doubt and cynicism pervades health care too.

Time and time again we hear calls to protect the poor 'victim' from the 'bad' system. Indeed, to read much of popular healthcare commentary, we seem to be locked in victim behaviour – some dispirited cavern in our psyche or souls (Snow & Willard, 1989) where we actually need to feel constantly oppressed. As Rinpoche again reminds us, 'Sometimes even when the cell door is flung open, the prisoner chooses not to escape.'

Perhaps we whinge so much and stay locked in our victimhood because at some level we need to. No matter how good the system gets, we still have some deeper need that comes from that dispirited martyristic part of ourselves to feel that it's 'their' fault. This seems to square with some of the worrying conclusions about the kind of people (us!) who come into nursing specifically and health care generally (Snow & Willard, 1989). Maybe we need to do as much work on ourselves, and our reasons for being in the work we have chosen, as acquiring more practical knowledge and skills, if we are to escape the 'land of shadow' (Plato, 1987, translated by Reed) and perceive a deeper reality that may be at work.

Blame the system? The system is a mere abstraction, a projection from our collective egos about how something should be in the world. As an ego projection, it is more concerned with issues of power and control than creativity and change. The system is simply a manifestation of ourselves. *We* – those who work in it, govern it and create it – are the system. Accepting this premise rais-es an intriguing and perhaps uncomfortable possibility. Changing the system is never really going to make much difference to people's lives unless we who are the system transform ourselves first. It is doubtful if that is achievable without a wholesale re-spiriting of who and what we are.

Holism and unholy work

Many studies have indicated high levels of suicide, stress and burnout among health professionals, as suggested in Chapter 2. Obvious factors involved are heavy workloads and the 'I can take it' culture in health care. The roots of the problem, however, go much deeper, as Snow and Willard's (1989) study was one of the first to indicate. The tendency to find identifiable solutions that we can use to fix a problem is a sweetly seductive approach, particularly if they re-inforce the victimhood of the carer in the face of the oppressive regime. Thus, in this view the roots of the problem lie external to ourselves – get the right workloads in place, provide a counselling service and some nicer managers, and it's sorted!

This fails to take account of other factors – some of which are more diffi-cult to take on board, because it means we have to look a little more deeply, and perhaps uncomfortably, at what is going on in ourselves. This strategy is doubly difficult because it risks blaming the victim – manna from heaven to the hard-nosed manager who would find it easier to blame the carer rather than examine and change the blameworthy situation in which they themselves are working.

Despite the common assertion in health care that we work in 'holistic ways', much of the writing on holism in the professional literature is in fact reduc-tionist. The bastardised mind-body-spirit version of holism in current parlance implies that we practise holism if we give a bed bath (body), refer the patient to a psychotherapist or social worker to sort out their problems (mind) and ask the chaplain to see them when we know their religion (spirit). We can apply this same sort of thinking to the systems in which we work, reducing our organisations and their problem-solving abilities to notions of getting the right bits in the right places and all will be well.

Holism has its roots in the Germanic *haelan* from which, as explained above, we derive our words 'hale', 'whole', 'hearty', 'healthy' and 'holy'. Healthiness is thus associated with feeling whole, and feeling whole is connected with the holy – sacredness and reverence for the world and what is in it, and a sense of connection with each other, our work and perhaps with a cosmic or divine order of things. The modern field of quantum physics has returned to the idea of this interconnected universe. Bohm (1973), a protégé of Einstein's, wrote of 'the interconnectedness of different systems that are not in spatial contact' and how we 'are led to a new notion of unbroken wholeness which denies the classical analysability of the world into separately and independently existing parts'.

We have not yet quite grasped the implications of quantum physics or the mystical views of a holistic universe. Holism is not about putting bits together, but about recognising that any impression of bits is mere illusion. Everything, absolutely everything, is connected, bound together in a coherent whole in which all those bits we see as parts are really intrinsic to a vast, orderly pattern. A true understanding of holism has profound implications for healing and health care. We are far more than the limited perceptions of human beings as separate biological entities.

EVERYTHING IS CONNECTED

Meanwhile, what has all this got to do with healthcare staff committing suicide? It means we need to be wary of getting into simplistic solutions of what is a highly intricate issue. We are not just victims, poor things, being beaten by a nasty system.

We come into health care with all kinds of drives and motives – from our childhood and so on – that make solutions to the suicide problem much more difficult than we might care to admit. Thus, blaming the bosses is too easy – what part are *we* playing in this great drama? What has got us so hooked into caring work and our identification with our roles that it sets us on a destructive path? If it's so bad, why not get the hell out of it? How *do* you get the 'hell' out of health care, if you see what I mean?

In my work for the Sacred Space Foundation, I lost count long ago of the numbers of staff who have come into retreat, depressed and traumatised by their experience in caring work. It is a crisis of meaning and personhood – the very stuff of spirituality. Believing we are nurses or doctors or whatever other role label we identify with (and not beings who happen to work in these roles), we become deeply attached to them. But when these roles get challenged – when we are made redundant or the subject of a complaint, for example, we can fall apart. An attack on our role, in this scenario, is an attack upon ourselves. It's personal – and it hurts. Investing our faith in a role can be problematic for us. Benn (2000) has neatly summarised the evidence that people with religiosity are more likely to be healthy, and this includes comforting notions that we belong to something that is yet greater than ourselves. Religious practices and spiritual beliefs (whether god-centred or not) do seem to help us live in the world with a little more equanimity. They help us let go of what Snow and Willard (1989) called 'superhood' – if we are all there is, then it's all down to us when it all goes pear-shaped. Identification with a role and an overweening attachment to it helps us to function at one level in the workplace and to know what to expect of each other. But if the role is 'me', it becomes fundamentally unhealthy for us.

I recall a post-burnout doctor as he left the Foundation. He said 'I used to say "I am a doctor" – now I know I am a human being who happens to work as a doctor.' Such a shift in consciousness, a realignment of the way he perceived himself and his roles in the world, helped him to approach his work with a healthy non-attachment from then on. It was not detachment, note, which suggests indifference or a kind of emotional protection and distancing from reality. Non-attachment means that we no longer identify with roles and functions and all the limiting, destructive baggage they can bring to us. Non-attachment helps us to see the bigger picture and approach suffering without the compulsion to fix everything, to feel bad when we cannot, to be 'super' at everything. Non-attachment means that we have made a shift within ourselves where we can come compassionately to be servants *in*, rather than compulsive servants *of*, our roles.

The Sacred Space Foundation, Emmers Farm, Sparket, Cumbria CA11 ONA
tel: 01768 486868, www.sacredspace.org.uk

CHAPTER 5

ON EMPTY TIGERS AND A ROARING SEA – INTENTION, PRAYER AND GETTING OUT OF THE WAY

The time and my intents are savage-wild,
More fierce and more inexhorable far
Than empty tigers or the roaring sea.

Romeo and Juliet, William Shakespeare

COMING TO THE CENTRE

It was one of those moments in life when the grand theories that we may teach others are tested – when the chickens come home to roost.

Recently, someone I love very much became very sick and distressed. It was not just the illness, but the loss of all the hopes and dreams from her previously healthy expectations that was so very painful to bear. I arrived at her home with my armoury of personal concerns and several decades of knowledge and skill in health care. My particular approach to healing, Therapeutic Touch (TT), was well known to her – and offered and accepted with hope.

TT practitioners are taught to 'centre' themselves (Sayre-Adams & Wright, 2001), a meditative state which helps them let go of their extraneous thoughts and to put aside attempts to 'make' things happen. They centre to get into an internal, peaceful, watchful place where they can simply be available to patients and clients in a loving and compassionate way that allows the person to trigger their own healing.

This time it was different. My centring techniques initially failed me. What would normally take only a matter of seconds took nearly a quarter of an hour. Why? Because my head was full of my own agendas. My natural human compassion and my overriding will that someone I love should be healed was in charge. It took what seemed like a lifetime to let go of all my 'stuff', realising that until I did so my capacity to be available to her in the most open and loving way would be blocked. Thoughts spun around in my head – 'I want you to get better, I want the bleeding to stop, I want to take your pain away . . .' These and other parts of my own will whirled around me like the icy winter wind that comes off the mountains where I live. I caught myself listing demands, praying, exhorting and specifying. Time seemed to stretch interminably before all this could settle down and I could come to a place of calm and openness that put all my own agendas to one side.

Never have I found it so difficult to do that which I so simply teach to others: to let go of our own expectations and wishes for what we deem the healing of the other to be, and rest with trust and intention for the healing to emerge. This time it struck home. This time, for a while at least, I wanted it sorted. No relaxed centring – just make her better!

This is not to deny that we all have these wishes for the wellness of others. But most practitioners seem to be caught up by them for much of their working lives. Our desire for the relief of suffering of others is inevitable, but it can also harm us. How can we balance those natural human connections, which may indeed motivate us to superhuman efforts, but may also drag us down into exhaustion and burnout (see Chapter 4) when we cannot let them go. How do we come into that secure place in ourselves, that place of understanding encapsulated in the lines of Julian of Norwich, where we can trust that 'all shall be well, and all manner of thing shall be well' (Doyle, 1983).

Bishop George Hacker (1998) notes, in his excellent treatise on healing from a Christian perspective: 'One of the signs of growth in the spiritual life is a deepening trust in God and the way in which he holds us in his hands.' Others from different belief perspectives might interpret that differently – as the inevitable beneficence of the universal will, the loving compassion of the cosmic consciousness, the human mind–body link shifting into harmony. Whatever our view, it can be immensely difficult to hold to that trust in the face of human suffering, especially when it concerns someone with whom we have a deep attachment. Hacker goes on to caution about 'badgering, not trusting God' when we want certain outcomes for others, while acknowledging that 'Most of us do not come to a place of such trust overnight, and sometimes there has to be a great deal of badgering before we reach that point.'

INTENTIONALITY

One of the most important qualities in the work of those who work with healing (and all healthcare practitioners do so to a greater or lesser extent) is that of our 'intentionality'. The practitioner must have a strong motivation to help or heal, yet is able to set aside their own particular wishes and desires for the other. Intentionality implies not only the will to help or heal but also a specific goal in mind – but the goal is to facilitate the interaction, rather than seeking to control its outcome. At the same time, there is a paradox here: one seeks health and healing yet gives up the expectation of a particular change happening. The meditative exercise of centring helps us to meet, acknowledge and lay to one side our own agendas. Many healthcare workers report that while working with patients they attempt to concentrate on dealing with what is before them rather than getting caught up in 'ifs' and 'maybes' – and this has some of that centring quality about it. Many other practitioners deliberately develop meditative and contemplative strategies as part of their work with patients in order to remain centred – present and ready for action with patients or clients, compassionate, yet non-attached to outcomes. They have often learned how emotionally bruising it can be when they do not take care of themselves in this way (see also Chapter 4).

The identification of intent is at least as important as the focus of the intent – perhaps more so. That is, in order to work with healing successfully, practitioners must acknowledge their motives. While intention to help patients achieve their maximum state of wellbeing is ideal, practitioners may also profit from trying to understand their desire to help.

In Rogers' (1970) holistic model, intent is addressed under her concept of acausality. In this model everything and everyone – all 'energy fields' – are interconnected. What each of us does directly affects everyone else. Therefore the results of what one does are affected by other conditions, for example the other people involved, the environment in which it's done, and so on. So it is possible to have intent to do something and yet for the effects to be quite different. The intent in playing billiards may be to shoot the ball, having it hit two others and have all three go into the pocket – but the results can be anywhere between that and none of them going in. The intent in turning a patient every hour may be to prevent pressure sores, but they may still occur. Perhaps the intention in health care should not be just about relieving symptoms, pain or anxiety but in creating 'wholeness' in the person. It is important to keep that intention of wholeness clear and then let go of desires for particular outcomes.

Inherent in this concept is the idea that by our thoughts, our focused consciousness, we influence the outcome of any interaction. And this is essentially a non-local phenomenon, i.e. something in our consciousness can affect the physical reality of another even though they may be separated from us at a great distance. One of the basic tenets of quantum physics is that we are not discovering reality, but participating in the creation of it (Sayre-Adams & Wright, 2001).

And quantum physics, or at least the theory of it, may offer us one explanation of how the conscious intention of one or more persons can affect the wellbeing of another when there is no physical connection between them. In TT, for example, physical touch does not necessarily take place, with the practitioner holding the hands often close to but some inches away from the body. Studies on non-local healing such as prayer and TT are producing some intriguing and controversial results. Can it be possible that one person's intention can possibly affect the physical state of another even though they are nowhere near each other? Jeanne Achterberg, currently conducting research in Hawaii (reports in press) has recently released information that is stunning in its implications. She is a fine example of a scholar who has applied rigorous scientific enquiry to an area that many would find difficult to research. Using an MRI scanner and a variety of different types of 'healers' and patient health problems, she has recorded startling images when 'distant healing' is happening. For the first time, changes in the patients' bodies at the time of healing have been rendered visible and measurable by the scanner. Cutting-edge research like this is throwing wide open the possibilities of scientific enquiry and at the same time giving us insights into the mystery that is healing.

IS PRAYER PART OF CARE?

Florence Nightingale (cited in Macrae, 1995) observed that

> It did strike me as odd, sometimes, that we should pray to be delivered from 'plague, pestilence and famine', when all the common sewers ran into the Thames, and fevers haunted undrained land, and the districts which cholera would visit could be pointed out. I thought that cholera came that we might remove these causes, not pray that God would remove the cholera.

Nightingale was an immensely practical woman but also a mystic (B Dossey, 1999); she saw no problem with the notion of prayer and taking practical action to relieve suffering. To her it was not either/or, but both. Her advice would seem quite sound. While much recent work on prayer and non-local healing offers some interesting, not to say startling, possibilities, it seems a little premature to throw away the pills and kneel down in church, temple or mosque instead.

Not long ago I was close to the end of one of those long shifts – you know, one of those kinds of days when every moment seems filled with deep labour. My colleague and I were in the ward office, about to go home, and making plans for the next day's teaching programme on TT.

The young doctor entered, slumped at the desk, buried his face in his hands and sighed, 'How can I tell her? The drugs don't work anymore.'

We looked at him, then each other, sat down and asked what the problem was, and the tears trickled down his face as he faced the thought of telling a young woman that the battle to save her was lost. The cancer, assaulted by pretty much everything in the medical armoury, was on the march again and this time it wasn't going to be stopped. 'There's nothing more I can do.' He repeated like some woeful mantra.

Eventually and nearly simultaneously, my colleague and I said, 'Oh yes there is – you can pray for her.' The look on his face said the rest. We'd had many discussions about the scientific basis and otherwise of the complementary therapies, and this time he obviously thought we'd flipped. He is a hard-nosed scientist – a randomised control trial for every treatment or he isn't interested.

It was because he is a scientist that we made the suggestion we did. There may be times when there is nothing more we can do, but that does not stop us from being with people, either offering them the loving comfort of our presence – sitting with them on their 'mourning bench' as Wolterstorff (1987) expresses it – or being with them in our consciousness, our prayers, our compassionate intention for their wellbeing, whatever that may turn out to be.

Prayer is one of the commonest ways that we express our spirituality. For many people (indeed most) whose spirituality is god-centred, prayer involves an attempt at direct communication with the divine, making a request that something might come about. We can, however, also simply think of prayer as entreating another for assistance or holding a conscious wish or desire for some event to occur. Prayer is a heartfelt request that something might *be*.

Thus prayer is definitely not the exclusive province of the religious. Anyone can focus their conscious intention, in the case of illness upon the wellbeing of another as well as oneself. But why bother? Isn't prayer just another flaky New Age idea or a return to the dark ages of superstition? Not if the scientific evidence is anything to go by. An increasing body of rigorous scientific investigation is now pointing to the effectiveness of prayer in the promotion of healing (space does not permit detailed mention of all the studies, but for good overall summaries see Benson, 1996; L Dossey, 1997a, 2001). Despite the complexities of studying prayer, or even understanding if and how it works, an accumulating body of compelling evidence suggests that there is something here that has long been neglected in mainstream health care.

Byrd's (1988) study, for example, sparked the imagination of many involved in health care and, indeed, scientists generally by illustrating some of the classic features of the effects of prayer, since replicated in many other studies. The patients prayed for in Byrd's work were statistically more likely to get better, had fewer medical interventions and complications, and lived longer than the control group. Byrd's work and that of others since indicate that patients who are prayed for are more likely to get well with fewer problems than those who are not – and the studies suggest that the religious backdrop has little influence.

One study in South Korea (Cha et al., 2001) found that the women who were prayed for were 24 per cent more likely to get pregnant than those who were not. Another carried out among 150 patients in a cardiac angioplasty unit in the

USA (Krucoff et al., 2001) found that those in the prayed-for group had 50 to 100 per cent fewer complications. Krucoff has attempted to replicate this study on a larger sample, but this time the results were indifferent. These studies are startling in their results, but such phenomena are not new. The distinguished physician Larry Dossey has probably done more than any other doctor to raise awareness of the significance of research in this field (L Dossey, 2001), highlighting how so many of the studies have been ignored, despite their scientific rigour.

Fasten your seat belt before reading the next paragraph, for this is *X Files* stuff. A recent study published in the *British Medical Journal* (Leibovici, 2001) has really set the cat among the medical pigeons, if the subsequent furious website correspondence and letters pages of the journal were anything to go by. Not only did prayer have an impact on patients with blood diseases, but also the effects were *retroactive* – the patients were prayed for in 2000, but their illnesses occurred in 1990-96! In other words, somebody praying for you in the future may affect your health status now. If this is mind-boggling, it's not surprising. It upends all our conventional notions of linear time and space, although to the quantum physicist or mystic the idea is perfectly feasible. To the latter, time is not linear and consciousness can affect things non-locally. Leibovici is not alone. Braud (2000) summarised the results of 19 studies where people attempted to influence a variety of living systems retroactively and he found ten to be statistically significant.

So, what is going on? Is God more likely to intervene if we ask? Are other phenomena at work? The studies cited above, up to the recent work of Achterberg, are indeed suggesting that something is going on that we do not fully understand. It may be divine intervention, it may be something in the consciousness of human beings that is able to connect with and affect other human beings that we cannot yet explain. Whatever the possibilities, this is the territory where science and spirituality are meeting.

The rising number of university departments dedicated to consciousness studies offers us some clues. If the idea of the divine is anathema to you, then you can see it from a different perspective. An increasing body of evidence is subverting the traditional notion (in the West) that consciousness is just a product of our brains. Consciousness appears to be non-local and is not governed by time and space. We do not so much contain consciousness as are held *in* consciousness. This is not a surprising notion to the modern scientific field of quantum physics, nor would it be to the mystics down the ages. Nor is it, surprisingly, to thousands of 'ordinary' people for whom the numinous experience has been a major event in their lives – a feeling of the oneness and interconnectedness of all things (Maxwell & Tschudin, 1996). A deeper understanding of consciousness may therefore be the key to understanding the phenomenon of prayer. On the other hand, you may be content to accept the religious explanation. Whichever the case, something seems to be going on, which suggests prayer might work and can affect health. Because of this, it is a territory worthy of further consideration and research.

The research, if intriguing, is by no means conclusive and we need much better assessment tools to find out what a patient's spiritual needs are before we offer help in this way (see Chapter 23). Most authors agree that prayer should only be offered in the light of this with consent, as with any other healthcare intervention, although Dossey (1997a) has wondered if we really need to ask consent to offer love. We also need to unpick our own agendas from it – praying in desperation or with demands for specific outcomes does not appear to be any more helpful. Simply praying that a person be made whole, or healed, or that suffering be relieved – whatever that form may take – may be all that is needed, while others such as Hacker (1998) have been more pointed, as suggested above. Certainly health professionals will need to gain a much deeper understanding of prayer and its impact than we generally have at present – pooh-poohing it as unscientific or irrational just won't do. If prayer works, and the debate still rages around that 'if', we are going to need much more imaginative ways of integrating prayer into normal practice if its benefits are to be available to patients, while avoiding the pitfalls of religious proselytising or even 'negative prayer'. In one study (cited by Dossey, 1997a) some 5 per cent of American Christians admitted to praying for harm to come to others!

However, it's not all one way. If the placebo effect works, there can also be a downside, what Hamer (2004) calls the 'nocebo' effect. His report on negative expectations of health, for example amongst people who are depressed or those who feel that God has abandoned them, raises some alarming concerns. Many of the studies on religiosity suggest positive benefits for health. But there can be a darker side. When we believe that we are not loved by God, or even worse that God has turned against us, or if we are atheist, simply feel hopeless, unloved or that there is no future for us, then we are more likely to get sick or die.

As the various studies suggest, it seems not to matter whether you are a Buddhist or a Christian, a humanist or a Hindu – something happens in prayer that seems to work and no belief system can lay claim to exclusive ownership (or denial) of it. But Florence Nightingale's quote above is apt. It's not a case of either work *or* prayer, but finding the benefits that come from both. As an old Islamic proverb says, 'Trust in God but tie your camel'!

Whatever is going on here – be it divine intervention or something about the nature of time and consciousness that we are only just beginning to scientifically explore, the implications are profound. Studies like those cited above are pushing at the boundaries of healthcare knowledge and if the evidence continues to mount we will have less and less excuse for ignoring it. The health service is, after all, supposed to be an 'evidence-based' system. We may never again be able to say, 'There's nothing more we can do.' It may be wondered how long it will be before we have prayer groups setting to work both inside and outside our hospitals, as has already happened formally in some US hospitals and as still occurs informally with local religious groups when someone gets sick. Mary Self (2001), a doctor who believes she was cured of her 'terminal' cancer through prayer, offers a fascinating example of the work of prayer in a religious community. This also raises some disturbing questions around prayer. Do people who have been prayed for and who do not get better feel let down or damned by God? Why do some get better and not others? Do those doing the praying feel that they have not prayed hard enough if the person does not improve? And what kind of capricious God is it that seems willing to help some and not others? Many profound practical and theological problems are raised in these prayer studies. It is also worth remembering that most of the studies are multi-denominational – no one form of prayer, Jewish, Christian, Islamic, etc. – has been found to be 'better' than any other. This is an exciting and fascinating frontier and, like all frontiers, it has opportunities but risks as well.

Healthcare practitioners want to relieve people's suffering or see an illness cured. It's a natural if limited human perspective, but it may be important also to remember that we cannot be sure of the meaning and purpose of suffering for another, or what healing for another precisely entails. Perhaps it is better when working with patients therefore to pay particular attention to staying centred, letting go of all our agendas and simply focusing on being with the other in a loving and compassionate way as we bring all of our attention, healthcare actions and intention upon them. Thus we can let go of ideas like, 'Let the heart pain go away' – such thoughts can be allowed to drift quietly into the background. It may be better to simply hold an intention for the other that they be healed, that they be whole – whatever that healing or wholeness might be for them.

In 2001 the devastating animal disease foot and mouth hit large swathes of the British countryside. My home in Cumbria is surrounded by farmland and normal life was governed for almost a year by severe isolation and infection control restrictions. A meditation group meets at my home monthly and we faced the possibility, as the outbreak was under way, that the meeting at that time would be the last for many months. Travelling around in rural areas became increasingly problematic and many rural people were shut off in their homes and farms in order to prevent the spread of infection. We sat in stillness and silence as usual, but one person suggested, 'Perhaps we could pray for the survival of the animals around us?' We are a multi-faith group, and prayer and meditation mingle freely. So we did.

And the livestock in my valley? Foot and mouth swept all before it, and for 50 miles around us not a cloven-hoof beast remained. Except for the three farms that border my house. But then, that probably was just coincidence, wasn't it?

Wait without hope

In the personal experience, which I have described on page 45, it took me some time to get myself into that centred place, to put aside my own will. It took not a little effort to recognise my (natural) will at work and to let it rest on one side – not to ignore it or suppress it; simply to acknowledge its existence and put aside my own hopes and expectations in order to be fully present. To get to a place which TS Eliot (1944) called waiting 'without hope, for hope would be hope for the wrong thing'.

However, does all this conflict with Hacker (1998) when he cautions that with prayers for healing:

> It is fashionable to tack the phrase 'if it be thy will' or something similar on to the end of a prayer. It may be that we genuinely do not know what is best for the person concerned, but often we do, or think we do, and if we really care about them then we need to ask plainly for what we want.

To do otherwise may 'introduce a defeatist element' into our prayers suggesting that we betray 'a lack of trust in God in that it shows a limited expectation of what he can do'. Is pulling back from specific wishes for another's wellbeing showing a lack of trust or such absolute trust that to ask for specifics is unnecessary? Perhaps both positions have some truth in them, whether our universe is god-centred or not. Prayer or entreaty to the deity may be seen to have different qualities of consciousness than the personal clearing out of the will through intention. Intention, underpinned by trust, seems to be the key factor at work. Doing what has to be done to help the other, holding an intention for wellbeing in one's heart for the other, may be all that is needed – and trust, however we hold or express it – is the vehicle that carries our intention to its fulfilment.

When intention hurts

I have spent years working with healthcare professionals in distress, and worked with them to help them let go of their fixed agendas and firmly held desires for specific patient outcomes. After all, it is these ties that can bind us into exhausting relationships with patients. Caught up in the drama of their suffering, which becomes our drama, we become burned out by the hurts and injustices and wrongs done to others (see Chapter 4). We can become attached to their suffering, and healthcare workers, if they are not very careful, can find themselves falling apart under the weight of such burdens (Ram Dass & Gorman, 1990).

Historically, professionals have responded to the risks of this kind of burnout by advocating a certain professional detachment or distance. I long ago lost count of the number of times I was told during my training, and since, 'not to get involved'. Latterly, we have seen a greater acceptance in orthodox health-care circles that partnership and 'being with' patients (Benner & Wrubel, 1989) is acceptable – with measures such as clinical supervision being advocated (Hawkins & Shohet, 1991) as a protective device for practitioners so that they do not get too caught up in patients' problems. Many would argue that such professional closeness has always existed among those who have practised in the complementary/alternative medicine (CAM) field, as Fulder (1996) suggests. Indeed, a recent issue of the *British Medical Journal* (2001) examined how the integration of CAM with orthodox medicine could help 'restore the soul' to medicine: 'Integrated medicine focuses on health and healing rather than disease and treatment. The patient is seen as a whole – complete with dreams, disappointments, stories, loved ones and enemies . . .' Such an approach requires doctors to see patients in a wholly (holy) different way and 'not just a biochemical puzzle to be solved' (Reilly, 2001).

However, the acceptance of CAM into mainstream care is no guarantee that it will become any more holistic than at present. It is just as possible for a CAM practitioner to get hooked on their particular health technology as an orthodox one. Getting 'lavender oil three times a day' added to the treatment sheet would not be a sign of a restoration of the soul of medicine or the success of integration. It would be a mark of failure.

The reductionist approach so prevalent in modern health care (encapsulated by the *BMJ*'s comments about the doctor 'only interested in elbows') is not going to be resolved if all we mean by integration is colonising some bits of the CAM field that come up to our standards of scientific scrutiny. The issue is not about whether we twiddle the patient's toes with a little reflexology or insert a new sort of heart valve. The technological intervention is only one aspect of the healing process, a conduit for some other, perhaps more significant, phenomenon to occur.

More and more evidence is pointing to the quality of the practitioner-patient relationship as the key factor in diminishing the stress of dis-ease, taking the immunosuppressive brakes off and releasing people's inherent self-healing capacity. Whether that comes from the healing 'energies' that so many CAM approaches adopt, or the neuropeptide flow observed in the leading work of Candace Pert (1997) and others, probably doesn't matter too much. Who we are – not what we do with people – seems to be just as important in healing the sick. When doctors and other carers are able to *be with* patients as well as *do to* them with equal presence and skill, then we will indeed have (re)discovered the soul of medicine.

Such a holistic approach is of real benefit to patients and may also help a lot of carers. A core difficulty of many carers who reach the crisis point of burnout and exhaustion is the breakdown of *relationships* with their colleagues and patients, and a loss of faith in their work through lack of ability and opportunity to work with real people and 'practise as I know it should be done'. Such difficulties are heightened by attachment to absolute outcomes for patients, and to treatments imbued with faith as rigid and binding as any dogma. They are exacerbated by senses of failure or defeat in the face of the disease onslaught or by the refusal of the patient to cooperate or get well.

CAM may help some doctors and others to get into right relationships and reconnect with their work and the people they seek to serve – good for their own souls as well as their patients'. But on its own, CAM is just a red herring, a straw clutched by a drowning person when all the while the lifeboat drifts nearby. Making CAM an add-on to the technological armoury of treatments will do nothing to halt the downward spiral of soulless medicine, unless the underpinning ethos of CAM is brought with it. Taken on its own, adoption of CAM may do no more to help the state of modern health care, and those who work in it, than the illusion cast by any other seductive quick-fix solution. A wholesale reappraisal of healing relationships is called for and that includes a deeper examination of the ways that carers can be so bound up in the healing processes of another that they become wounded as a result. Learning to pull back a little on our own will and our ideas for patients; to apply our knowledge and technical know-how yet also stand back from becoming over-attached to specific outcomes; to practise with compassionate non-attachment; to refocus our prayerful intention; to trust in the possibility of a deeper will and purpose at work – these and other issues are worthy of closer exploration by those involved in health care.

CHAPTER 6
DEEP LISTENING – GETTING OUT OF THE WAY EVEN MORE

Such harmonious madness
From my lips would flow,
The world should listen then – as I am listening now.

'Ode to a Skylark', PB Shelley (in Gardner, 1989)

WHAT IS HEARD MAY NOT BE WHAT IS SAID

When the rain comes to Uluru, red turns to green. This ancient sacred heart of Australia (named Ayer's Rock by colonising Europeans) sits in the very centre of the continent's red desert.

But unseasonal big rains had come. The desert bloomed and became lush with vegetation, the once arid air was full of the sweetness of rare flowers, humid and heavy, vibrant with the sound of insects. Like so many spiritual seekers from the West who had cast off the shackles of their established religion, I had danced for a little while around the edges of the belief systems of indigenous peoples. And I can see why some of them despise us for it. Materially wealthy, we satiate our spiritual poverty by sucking on the traditions of others who we see as possessing something we have lost. In so doing, we often look for the best bits we like and put off the bits we don't, unwilling to really commit and do the hard work that is an element of all spiritual practice.

My dalliance with these traditions lasted a few years before I finally found Home in the most unexpected of places, but that is another story. Meanwhile, here I was in the middle of the land of Oz, with my very own wizard, or equivalent thereof. He was an aboriginal elder, leader, shaman and healer. Twinkly eyed and leather skinned, with an air of profound patience with yet another Westerner about to rip off his culture. We took tea in a plush hotel, both feeling out of place in the kind of construction designed to keep you safely walled off from the reality of nature – all glass and air conditioning and the distractions of pools and bars and carefully manicured gardens.

We talked until the setting sun drowned the land in purple, and we walked across a patch of scrub now heavy with scent. He stepped over the bones of a long-dead lizard and spoke of the aboriginal tradition of 'pointing the bone': essentially, holding a 'magic' bone in one hand while pointing it at the victim and repeating a curse – the person had to see and hear what was going on. This was a sort of negative prayer. The victim would usually be so terrified and culturally attuned to believe in the effects of the bone pointing that whatever the curse was about would invariably happen – become sick or die. We laughed a little about this and he said, 'That must seem very strange to you; I don't suppose that sort of thing happens in your country.'

I thought about this and, yes, there's more than enough tradition in Europe of cursing and it has not died out. It's just more subtle. True, I haven't seen many nurses in Penrith waving chicken wings at their 'difficult' patients. But there are other ways that it works. In our empowering, knowledge-sharing, everything-upfront culture, I sometimes wonder if *all* information giving is helpful. The patient asks, 'How long have I got to live?' and we might say, 'Six months', and wonder why some of them die in about that time. If we are not careful about the way we give bad news, it can become a self-fulfilling prophesy. What used to be called mind over matter is now more scientifically validated as the PNI (psychoneuroimmunology) effect. Candy Pert has led the way in her research in this field (Pert, 1997), showing how our emotional state has a direct impact upon our physical bodies – our beliefs affect our cells.

Consider then the impact upon a patient diagnosed with a serious illness who asks about her prospects, if someone knowing the likely course of the disease says, 'Well, after five years only 10 per cent survive.' Now with a subtle change of emphasis and tone, how might the emotional response be changed? 'Well, yes, it's serious, but you know 10 per cent of people have been known to survive this disease.' The former is the counsel of despair, the second of hope, and the emotional impact of either may affect the outcome.

We may not point bones anymore, but in modern health care, if we are not careful with our words, we can deliver a curse as damning as any mediaeval witch or aboriginal shaman.

THE SOAP OPERA OF THE SLEEPING SPIRIT

Words and how we speak and receive them are full of power. Yet so often we speak without really discerning the impact upon the listener; or what we think we are saying can have layers of spin applied by the listener depending on mood, culture and a myriad other factors. A doctor told me her story:

> *I'm worn out. I feel like I'm caught up in vast episode of* Eastenders *and can't get out of it. The play just keeps going on and on and there isn't even a commercial break. Everybody is speaking, but nobody is really listening. And it's not even as if the words are real: it's like I'm an actor in one of these plays and I'm saying these words, but it's the actor speaking and the words don't mean anything because they're not really* my *words. And when somebody speaks to me they're not using their words either and what they hear is words that aren't really me, so nobody is really listening or talking to each other at all, and I just can't stand it anymore.*

This young woman had come to me in our retreat (the Sacred Space Foundation) in Cumbria for some guidance on how to get out of the stress and burnout she was in. Interestingly, the pain of her situation was also waking her up to the reality of her everyday working relationships. Her symptoms are typical. The world starts to look and sound different, and in this instance she was reacting (painfully) to the shallow interactions that she now perceived in her daily life.

Eastenders is a popular soap opera on TV in the UK; it has its soapy counterparts all over the world, and in all soaps the essential plots and characters are the same, dressed up in different outfits and playing against different backdrops or using different words. The subtext of themes is universal, seductive and repellent simultaneously. Work, life and relationships in them are all about power, treachery, manipulation and mistrust. Love (when not distorted as possession), happiness, joy and connection are rare – they don't seem to make good storylines apparently. Our attention seems more easily engaged by the superficial, the dramatic, the cut and thrust of constant attack and defence in a myriad of forms and situations. Problems are solvable only by angry outbursts, walkouts or violence. The characters speak, but nobody really listens. What is heard is filtered through the recipient's own agendas, editing and judgements.

JUST MISSING

Is it possible to go beyond superficial perceptions and become aware of what is really being said behind the words? What most of us experience at work and at home are endless conversations where we don't quite connect with what is really going on between us. The boss tells the office staff that she wants to do some (what she sees as reasonable) restructuring to make the service more efficient. They hear threats to their livelihoods, feel the despair of possibly more interviews, get anxious and competitive with colleagues, feel angry and powerless at decisions being made without a sense of involvement, connection or understanding. The gap between what is said and what is heard can be as wide and deep as the Grand Canyon and equally tough to traverse. Caught up in our roles, we can come to really believe we are the part we play; but when we live in roles, we speak in them too and the connection between people remains forever superficial, artificial, like actors in dialogue – real people are not speaking to each other.

Entrapment in this way 'alienates us from one another: a social worker and juvenile offender just miss; a nurse and patient seem worlds apart; a priest and parishioner so distant, so formal. What otherwise would be a profound and intimate relationship becomes ships passing in the night' (Ram Dass & Gorman, 1990, page 125). Thus countless situations arise in relationships where we 'just miss'. The potential for healing and compassion, for connection with another human being, shorn of our own ego's priorities of control or defending from fear, and so on, gets lost in our soap-opera dialogues.

The nurse sees it as a simple test – an electrode here, a machine there. The patient says, 'That's alright, I'm not worried. Do you think there's a problem with my ticker then?' A reassuring platitude from the nurse glides over the question. What the patient is really saying is:

> *Actually I'm quite worried, all kinds of things are tumbling through my head, if I turn out to have a heart problem and there must be a problem if I'm here and what's that beeping sound going off for and is this going to get worse or better and how the hell will I tell my wife, and the office manager will go apeshit if I go off sick and I'm really scared and I'm pissed off trying to make like I feel all right and why can't you SEE that I'm not alright, you're supposed to be a bloody nurse and why don't you pay attention to me instead of that damn machine . . .*

And the nurse carries on because:

> *If I stop for a moment and really pay attention to this guy the whole damn queue will just get longer and I don't have the time to deal with his anguish and I'm not sure I know what to say anyway and, God, I need a cup of coffee and that bloody nurse is going to be off again and no matter what I say or do I can't seem to get her to be more responsible and doesn't she realise what a burden she is to the rest of us with her swinging the lead and, Christ, my back aches and I'm knackered and really shouldn't have had that extra vodka last night and will Sheila really remember to go to the bank today, why don't you leave me be, mother, and let me get on with my own life . . .*

So much of what is going on in modern health care is governed by superficial listening. Meetings where big decisions are being made are usually great power games. Rarely is there opportunity for silence and reflection, to establish right relationship, to perceive what is really the best outcome, liberated from the shackles of our own agendas to be in control, to have our own way, to impose our own image upon the world. An organisational culture addicted to power nurtures this, but we also often lack the insight to see a better way.

DEEP LISTENING

Preoccupied with our own stuff, trying to listen while at the same time assessing and framing a reply, are barriers to deep listening. We can't do all these at the same time as *really* paying attention to someone in need. Thus in countless situations we just miss, and an opportunity for human connection is lost. Listening at this deep level does not come easily and is rarely arrived at simply by life experience. It takes courage – to halt a conversation and ask for a moment's silence to reflect, to ask a meeting to hold a space while a prayer is offered for guidance and clear thinking, to learn approaches such as meditation, which can offer us insights into who we are and what makes us tick.

Holden recognises the toughness of this task, for to deeply pay attention to another we have to get ourselves out of the way, yet 'underneath the masks we all wear, everyone feels lacking or flawed to some degree' and typically we 'fear to investigate these feelings too closely lest you become overwhelmed and lose the ability to appear that you have it all together' (Holden, 2002). Holden goes on to point out how we project these feelings on to others, by trying to fix them, control them or receive communications as if they are an attack upon ourselves – an attack to be robustly defended. Thus we rarely listen deeply because we are already busy with our own interior plans, assessing what to do and how to respond or keep control of the situation. It is not possible to listen fully when we are already engaged in preparing a reply. Communications fall into games of emotional ping-pong, with the players at a safe distance never really connecting with each other.

The solution is to encourage the evolving of more well-rounded human beings who can see beyond the masks that we present to each other, and this can only be done, in the view of Holden and many other spiritual teachers, by adopting a commitment to spiritual practice and expansion of our consciousness that connects us to the deep peace and safety that lies in our very essence, our souls. Without this spiritual maturity we are afraid to operate other than behind our masks and roles, for who on earth would be left if we let them drop even for a little while? To 'switch off the demanding self' (Pym, 1999) so that you can pay close attention and witness the drama at play requires, for most of us and our workplaces, a wholly (holy!) different way of being in the world. There is little evidence that our healthcare organisations actively engage in promoting this spiritual maturity of their workers, yet I suspect the investment in this support would have huge payoffs, in financial and human terms, in a dramatic reduction of errors and complaints that currently are costly in every sense of the word.

When we can confidently set aside our ego agendas, we can get ourselves out of the way. This enables the listener to:

> Totally switch off his or her own views for the duration of the 'listen'. By doing so he is able to give his total attention to the speaker. In the process he or she will have a brand new experience: by not interrupting or arguing he will hear things that he has never heard before. The speaker too will have a brand new experience. He will be aware that he is being heard by someone who is not going to come back to him with a reply, criticism or opposition. And not only is he heard, he hears himself.
>
> (Pinney, cited in Pym, 1999)

As Pym suggests, informed by his Quaker beliefs, it is quite possible to train people to listen in this way and this is coupled with attention to spiritual awakening. Margaret Guenther, in her excellent treatise *Holy Listening* sees the importance of learning to 'pay attention, to listen to what is not being said (or to what is being said but minimised,)' and to learn the art of 'waiting' and 'asking the right questions' rather than having the right answers (Guenther, 2002). Giving space to speak enables the person to feel heard – and simple techniques like the Native American 'talking stick' approach for example (the person who holds the stick must be listened to without interruption) can be remarkably effective in offering not only time to speak, but also time to listen. The use of silence, waiting, getting the self out of the way and ensuring the (sacred) space for the other to speak enables a deeper quality of listening to take place, which can truly promote healing, understanding, compassion and connection.

I guess to many the thought of working or living like this is pie in the sky, but I work with some adventurous organisations and people who are beginning to integrate these approaches into their work and lives. As suggested in Chapter 2, more enlightened organisations are indeed paying attention to the spiritual support and awakening of their staff. I work with one where it is common practice to begin each board meeting with a moment of prayer, reflection and silence; to pause the meeting and hold a silence if agreement is not clear or conflict is developing. That same organisation actively promotes policies of spiritual growth and support for its staff.

It can be done, and it feels so much better than being stuck in the eternal soap opera. Take the next opportunity to watch one of the soaps. It may be just a confection, a drama, a temporary distraction, but as the good doctor cited earlier suggests, for a lot of people that's real life, and it hurts.

CHAPTER 7

IF GOD IS ALL – DOES THAT INCLUDE MEASLES? REFLECTIONS ON DUALISM AND ONENESS

The amount of happiness that you have depends on the amount of freedom that you have in your heart. Freedom here is not political freedom. Freedom here is freedom from regret, freedom from fear, from anxiety and sorrow. I have arrived, I am home, in the here, in the now.

Thich Nhat Hanh, 1993

HOME FROM HOME

Thich Nhat Hanh's offer of resting peacefully in the here and now, at home, can seem almost dreamlike when we are caught up in the everyday world with thoughts endlessly racing between past, present and future. Yet it seems to be the essence of being healed and of the quality of the one who works in health and healing. So, as people gathered from all over the world in Cumbria last April, for the conference on Spirituality and Health, I found myself reflecting on home and what it means to us, and of the longing for home, the very source of it being not just the house or country where I live. This longing for home is so beautifully captured in the words of Rumi, who speaks of his soul being 'from elsewhere' and the realisation that he exists in this reality like a drunk in a tavern, lost and disorientated, awaiting the one who brought him there to take him 'home' (Rumi, 1997). By 'home' he refers to his place of origin in his Beloved, God, the Absolute, the source from which he wandered and to which he knows he will return. The place of safety, indeed the only place of safety where he can truly be at peace. Meanwhile his heart longs to be in that place of 'home' now, a place where he rests completely and lovingly in this moment – regardless of where he is in space and time in ordinary reality.

I am remembering now a time as a child when I came home after my first day at school. I had been heartbroken to be left in that classroom, but coming back to our house late afternoon, curled up in my chair next to the window and listening to the sound of my mother clattering pots in the kitchen; the smell of apple pie cooking – home.

For most of us a particular place means home – the place of family, of familiar things, of shelter and security. We construct in the outer world a place that resonates with our inner longing to be at peace, a place to rest among the familiar, which is safe and known to us. As Rumi suggests, there is a deeper meaning to home, a longing for our source, our origin to which no earthly home can ever compare and which, consciously or unconsciously, we are forever seeking. The ache in Rumi's heart for home could seem despairing or hopeless – for it is forever out of reach, somewhere else in the distance, perhaps at death. But Rumi, in his other works, as in the writings of all the great mystics, indicates a more hopeful tone. That home can be found in the here and now, not dependent upon a particular house or town or country, but a profound way of being in the world where we are richly connected to all that is – to our Source, to God, to the Absolute, whatever we perceive this to be. When we come home in this sense, then we do not depend on a particular place or situation to be at home, for we are forever at home within ourselves. Everywhere in external reality is then home.

Feeling spiritually homeless is reinforced if we live in a dualistic view of the world, where for example there is God and not-God, good and evil, light and dark. For those of us who work in health care this is primarily manifested in our approach to disease – 'the battle against cancer', 'the war against AIDS', 'the struggle against old age' – and so on. Our language encapsulates a separatist world view that encourages a state of endless struggle, and there are consequences for us both personally and collectively if we stick with this view.

ONE ON ONE

There is a Sufi saying (Sufism is the mystical school of Islam) that 'It is easy to know one, it is easy to know two, but to truly understand that one and one are two we must also know "and".' It is the mysterious binding force, to which this proverb alludes, that takes away the notion of separateness, where struggle is dissipated in the knowledge to which both mystics and modern physicists point – all is one. All the great faiths have words in their sacred books that offer us this wisdom. Guru Nanak, the founder of the Sikh faith, made a pilgrimage to Mecca. Sitting in the street, a passer-by remonstrated with him that it was an insult to sit with the soles of his feet pointing towards the Kaaba – the most holy shrine at Mecca. 'Show me where God is not,' replied Guru Nanak, 'and

I will point my feet there!' In the Qur'an we read that 'He is all that the heavens and the earth contain' (Qur'an, translated by Dawood, 1991) and in the Old Testament of 'the God who maketh all' (Ecclesiates 3: 11). The Buddhists speak of enlightenment being the recognition that 'the knower and the known are one' (the Dhammapada, translated by Mascaro, 1973); the Hindus say 'God is all' (the Baghavad Gita, translated by Mascaro, 1962) and suggest that 'everything is pervaded by the divine' (the Upanishads, translated by Easwaran, 1988). Christians repeat the Apostles' Creed, which states that God 'is the maker of all things visible and invisible' and find in many texts of the New Testament the assertion of a God where 'all things were created through him and for him' (Colossians 1: 15–20). The great Jewish invocation, the Schma, reminds believers that there is no duality but that 'the Lord thy God is One', while the Tao 'is the source' which has 'all things within it' (Tao Te Ching, translated by Streep, 1994). A pagan chant affirms 'Oh great spirit, earth and sky and sea, you are inside and all around me.' Thus, in all belief systems, despite the many references to battles between good and evil in all their forms, we find the counter-affirmation that at a deeper level everything is one – a 'dvaita', as it is called in Hinduism, non-duality.

SEPARATION IS AN ILLUSION

We live in a world of separation and it can be a tall order to accept, when faced with the suffering child, that the divine is not only in the child but in the measles as well. In the *Brothers Karamazov* (Dostoyevsky, 1880), Ivan the atheist provides a cogent argument against his theistic brother that there can be no God worthy of worship. For if he allows the innocent to suffer, having made all the creation, then he is unworthy of worship because he will not intervene. If, on the other hand, God is only good and does not always prevail against evil, then he is equally unworthy of worship through not being all-powerful. Modern theologians such as Vardy (1992) explore this theme further, and still reach dualistic conclusions of divided forces at work in the world. This centuries-old debate seems to be missing the point if we take a leap of the imagination into another possibility that suffering is grace (Ram Dass, 2000) – the very fuel of the fire of creation by which we strip away illusions of ordinary reality and come into a different level of consciousness. It is here, for those of us who work with the diseased and dis-eased, that the healing emerges. The sickness may continue (i.e. there is no 'cure') or indeed the person may die, but it is possible to die healed. It is worth remembering that healing, hale, whole, holy and home all come closely related from the same linguistic roots. And healing is more than a shift in bodily state; it is a shift of consciousness that comes when we see through the limited dualistic veils of the battle between sickness and disease, and break through into another realm where 'I am not my body, I am not my disease' – the realm where my deepest self, my essence, my soul is infinite, ever present, in perfect union with all that is.

And coming to this state of consciousness is not without price, for it is 'a condition of complete simplicity costing not less than everything' (Eliot, 1944). It is tough soul work, for as Eliot goes on to write:

> You must go by a way wherein there is no ecstasy.
> In order to arrive at what you do not know
> You must go by the way of ignorance.
> In order to possess what you do not possess
> You must go by the way of dispossession.
> In order to arrive at what you are not
> You must go through the way in which you are not.

Faced with the suffering of the sick it is tempting to lapse into the dualistic battle of opposing forces. Indeed, it seems unreasonable to do otherwise. Like motherhood and apple pie, freedom from disease is so self-evidently good that to argue against it puts us beyond the pale of being rationally human. Further, does this mean that we simply lie down and roll over in abject surrender in the face of sickness? Do we not act to treat disease? Of course we do, for to do otherwise would be to lapse into the dualism of denial as well. Action there is, but it is action deeply rooted in the awareness of all that is in this very moment, not just the disease as an entity with a life of its own. This is the realm of the effective healer, therapist, spiritual counsellor – to be with people in their suffering to find meaning, purpose and perhaps an expanded awareness or consciousness about their ill health. This is a coming home, when we stand back and look at our suffering and say 'Oh, how could it have been otherwise!', for here lies home, the place of peace, and it is a peace that 'passeth all understanding'.

If it is part of our role, as those who work with the sick and the dying, to play some part in the transcendence of suffering, it is equally part of our role not to deny the actions we can take in practical terms to relieve or prevent it. The burnishing of the soul that comes with our own suffering may bring us to some point where we are far more available to others who suffer, not in an exhausting co-dependent, battle-weary way, but from a place of helping where we are both doing and resting within ourselves. We act from a different place of consciousness, where we do what must be done, but from a place of deep stillness within. When we are not in this place of deep peace within, thereby lies the way of burnout and disconnection from self (see Chapter 4). And in being thus with ourselves and others, maybe, just maybe, that presence may help the other in their own onward, inevitable march home. The purpose of this soul work, from the 'healer's' perspective, is therefore not to isolate us from the human experience, but to plunge us ever more deeply into it.

The holistic, mystical perspective of being part of all that is, encourages us not to see ourselves as separate from anything. This shift of consciousness away from dualism helps us to see more clearly what is really going on, and enter the affray of illness 'but with peace in our hearts' (Thich Nhat Hanh, 1993).

I am reminded here of Harry, a patient I have written about in Chapter 18, and the shock of an experience of being with him in such a way that I did not feel separate from him. And, moreover, 'seeing' that despite his terrible physical and mental health problems, at some deeper level, I 'knew' he was absolutely OK – and he 'knew' it too. Vaughan and Walsh (1988) write of this viewpoint where

> . . . the sickness and suffering that seem inescapable from our egocentric perspective are recognised as illusions, incapable of harming our true Self in any way. All suffering is seen as but a dream. It follows that healing sickness and pain involves awakening from our collective dream and remembering who we really are. This awakening is known in various traditions as salvation, satori, liberation, or enlightenment. It does not necessarily involve changes in our physical circumstances because our pain and sickness, and even our bodies, are part of a dream. We need not seek to change our true nature, which is actually unchangeable. Rather we need only recognise, remember, and awaken to it, and the nightmare of suffering ceases to control us.

ONLY CONNECT

Without the level of connection with our deepest truth that Vaughan and Walsh describe, those of us who work in the healing and helping professions, or for that matter anyone who seeks to help another, are limited in the extent to which we can be truly available to those in need. We risk falling into the duality of the battle with dark and light, with the disease, the distress, whatever form it takes, as a worthy opponent to be defeated. What modern thinkers like Vaughan and Walsh and the great spiritual texts down the ages have offered us is a different perspective – there is no battle, for there is no enemy, for both exist only as part of the dream. When we wake up and rest at home in the true nature of reality, the exhausting conflict with disease disappears.

My work at the Sacred Space Foundation, where we offer retreat and recuperation facilities for carers who are burned out, has taught me many things, not least that that old chestnut 'burnout' is commonly exacerbated among carers who are caught up in the grand drama between good and evil – with physical, psychological, spiritual or social dis-ease being a force to be attacked.

The impact upon the carers is to spin them off ever more into the cycle of burnout (Wright & Sayre-Adams, 2000; Glouberman, 2002) and to keep them remote from the real comforting contact that the dis-eased person so needs. When we see ourselves in a dualistic world, we separate ourselves from the creation and from each other to a greater or lesser extent. There is no compromise here; separation from source also separates us from others.

In this model, the patient or client becomes a problem to be fixed. Arthur Frank (1991), in his reflections on his own illness, illuminates this sense of disconnection that the professionals can reinforce.

> To be professional is to be cool, and management orientated. Professional talk goes this way: a problem has come up, more serious than we thought, but we can still manage it. Here's our plan; any questions? Hearing this talk, I knew full well that I was being offered a deal. If my response was equally cool and professional, I would at least have a junior place in the management team. I knew that as patient choices go it wasn't a bad deal, so I took it. I was even vaguely complimented.
>
> I did not know the cost of taking that deal. Experiences are to be lived, not managed. The body is not to be managed, even by myself. MY body is the means and medium of my life; I live not only in my body but also through it. No one should be asked to detach his mind from his body and then talk about this body as a thing, out there.

All dis-ease brings with it a grieving, a mourning, a loss of some sort – of security, certainty, health, power, beauty, love. Those who grieve from whatever cause, however great or small, demand a certain way of being from their carers and comforters. Walterstorff (1987), in his lament for a lost son, further accentuates the sense of disconnection from helpers when they are busy being professional, or trying to fix things, or caught up in their own grand drama of the unending struggle for triumph over distress:

> If you think your task as comforter is to tell me that really, all things considered, it's not so bad, you do not sit with me in my grief, but place yourself off in the distance away from me. Over there, you are of no help. What I need to hear from you is that you recognise how painful it is. I need to hear from you that you are with me in my desperation. To comfort me, you have to come close. Come sit beside me on my mourning bench.

When we are unable or unwilling to sit upon the mourning bench alongside someone, we set ourselves apart from them. And we risk becoming Job's comforters. In the Bible, Job is beset by all manner of afflictions, but his situation is worsened by a series of friends who endlessly advise him or drown him in platitudes. If we get caught up in the patient's suffering, we risk forever trying to manage the problem or advise on, or fix it (and really seeking to make ourselves feel better in the bargain!) instead of sitting beside the person on their mourning bench and following Job's pleading advice:

> *Listen to what I am saying; that is all the comfort I ask of you.*
>
> Job 21: 1–2

Being with people in this deeply connected way does not lessen the actions we need to take to help and heal, nor does it lessen our witnessing of it. But the action and the witnessing come from a place of compassion within ourselves. Resting in the home and wholeness of our own self and awareness of a deeper level of reality, perhaps the real reality, we can act but without the burning-out energy of the battleground or the disconnection from the other in their suffering, for indeed there is no 'other' at all.

Some time ago, I found my own homecoming coming closer (though I see myself right now very much as 'work in progress') when I revisited the forgiveness of my parents. We all have our childhood wounds and I no less than others. I found a certain healing came some time ago when I learned to forgive my parents for those wrongs. It was a step along the way, but it was years later that I realised how much further there was to go. Forgiveness was not about a kind of condescending letting go of past wrongs, but a heartfelt realisation that there was indeed no 'wrong' at all. My parents and all they were and are to me have been absolutely perfect to bring me to this point, as I have been their perfect son. In some karmic web that seems a little vague to me now and difficult to pin down in words, I came to an awareness of that perfect unfolding, and with that came a great release. The energy we sometimes put into forgiving is released when we transcend even the illusions of right and wrong (*A Course in Miracles*, Anon, 1975).

Caught up in pain and suffering, it can seem a tall order to see forgiveness in this light, but it is perhaps the role that is demanded of all those who seek to help and heal, helping by the nature of our presence at home in ourselves, being the sacred space in which the wounded one's own healing can emerge. My own coming home has profoundly influenced the way I work with those who are dis-eased and diseased; I trust for the better. My long walk through 30 years of nursing offers a vista down the winding road along which I have travelled, while the road ahead seems forever veiled in mystery. But being at home makes you free of the fear of the unknown, for the known is home, beyond which everything is just fine.

When we work from Home, we can participate ever more fully in the relief of the suffering of others, and perhaps also stand back and witness the wonder of its unfolding. When we connect more deeply with the oneness of all, such an approach lifts us out of the battlefield of the sick room, out of the exhaustion and seduction of ego superhood that leads to burnout, out of the swampy lowlands of pity, past sympathy and into deep compassion – where you feel and know that everything is OK. As Mother Julian (cited in Doyle, 1983) wrote to remind us (re-mind us):

> *All is well,*
> *And all shall be well,*
> *And all manner of thing shall be well.*

CHAPTER 8

SOCKS, SILENCE AND STILLNESS
– REFLECTIONS ON THE
SANCTUARY OF MEDITATION

Their strength is to sit still.
Isaiah 30: 7

MOTHER AND MEDITATION

A conference gathering in the beautiful setting of Worth Abbey in southern England was set to explore the connection between healing and meditation. Like all good conference speakers I had arrived fully prepared for what I was going to say – honest! – and as I walked the labyrinth (a meditative spiralling pathway that aids reflection, prayer and contemplation; see Wright & Sayre-Adams, 2000 for a full description) seeking inspiration, for some reason all I could think of was my mother. She died 30 years ago and my memories of her seem few and thin now. It was not a family filled with intimate sharings and loving expressions; quite the reverse in fact. It was poor, working class; and you just got on with things. Anything personal was firmly buttoned up, only emerging perhaps at moments of fiery familial rages interspersed with long periods of the dull and the everyday and unmemorable.

So I was thinking of my mother and deeply aware of an intimate moment, a rare event I guess, when I was maybe seven or eight years old. I was sat on the floor at her feet in front of a roaring coal fire. She was silently in the midst of one of her regular rituals – the darning of socks. I remember those socks – hand knitted, made of hard grey wool reaching from feet to knees. I seemed to spend a lot of my childhood endlessly pulling them up. The wool stretched and they would always slip down to my ankles (unless a piece of elastic tied below the knees was used, which then seriously challenged the circulation of the

70

lower limb and made those woolly fibres itch all the more). 'Pull your socks up' was a regular roar of admonition from teachers and parents. It was an order literally to tidy yourself up by raising the socks to the knees, and metaphorically to remind you to work harder and get yourself organised.

But back to my mother: I was caught up in her silence and intensity. She was utterly focused on what she was doing, skilfully weaving thread and needle across gaping holes stretched over the wooden mushroom. There was a sharpness and clarity in her eyes, and for a moment there seemed to be absolutely nothing else existing in the world but the sound of the fire and the drift of her hands and her sharp steady gaze. 'What are you doing, mum?' I asked. (I recall how thunderous my words sounded in the stillness.) 'I'm making them better,' she answered. And the silence returned.

JUST HERE, NOW

Three and a half decades later I found myself talking about that very moment in the conference. I don't remember my mother ever using the word 'meditation'; she probably would not have known what it was. But she was certainly a meditator – utterly present in the moment, aware and responsive to her surroundings, yet all else was set aside as she simply sat in silence and darned. She was working and moving with skill and attentiveness. Nothing else was happening. She was just darning, making my socks 'better'.

A friend of mine was in hospital a few years ago and was desperately sick; indeed his life was in danger. He was married to a nurse, but as a non-nurse had thus far spent much of his married life studiously avoiding anything to do with nursing. We were having a heated discussion over the nature of nursing one evening over dinner (yes, sad I know!). It was long after his recovery, although he remains disabled to this day. He came out with one of the most profound insights about nurses, and other carers come to that, that I have heard from any layman. 'Steve,' he said, 'You guys have got it all wrong. There's only two types of nurses – the "glassy-eyed" and the "clear-eyed". The glassy-eyed ones came into his room, did all the nursing, seemingly as good as any other, 'but you could tell by the look in their eyes, no matter what they were saying to you or you to them, that they weren't really *with* you.' Such nurses and other healthcare practitioners are like the people you can meet at a party. You strike up a conversation, but you can tell by that glazed look in their eyes that they are not really interested in what you have to say – they are already thinking of what they want to tell you or have already moved on in their minds to wanting to talk to someone else.

He went on to talk about 'clear-eyed' nurses, who were 'absolutely present' for you. You could tell again by the look in their eyes – so clear, so attentive –

that nothing else was going on with them. They weren't thinking about the next job or what they did the night before. They were just right there for you, right there.

The capacity to 'be here now' (Ram Dass, 1971; Ram Dass & Gorman, 1990) for somebody has a meditative quality to it, an approach to caring where our own agendas and mental 'busyness' are set aside so that we can be fully attentive to the other. The best carers, of whatever sort – doctors, nurses, chaplains, social workers and the rest – are like my mother when darning socks – just being present and doing what needs to be done with full attentiveness and awareness. People feel better around such carers and, like my friend, when feeling better they are more likely to get better. He made another interesting observation; that his clear-eyed nurses were just as busy as the others, but it was something about the grace of their presence that made the difference. This supports my contention that a therapeutic relationship may not be dependent on time and the opportunity to get to know someone deeply; it may depend more simply on who we are, our capacity to be a 'presence' that is utterly attentive to the other (Benner, 1984). Not just doing, but being, determines the quality of the therapeutic encounter, however brief. The work of the expert carer is not just built on professional knowledge and skills; it is also dependent on understanding the immense healing power of our uncluttered selves – and that is a spiritual path requiring spiritual practices. Modern professional education pays much attention to the former. The latter is still a barely explored territory.

TO MEDITATE IS TO HEAL

Visualisation, imagery, chanting, journeying, contemplation, prayer – these and more are words loosely and often confusingly used to describe meditation. If we have a problem we are often advised to meditate upon it, implying a goal-oriented sitting in silence. But meditation with a purpose is something of an oxymoron. For to meditate is paradoxically to come to a place of purposelessness – simply to be, present and aware in the moment. Eileen Caddy, one of the founders of the famous Findhorn Foundation, once said to me, 'Prayer is when I talk to God, meditation is when I listen.' Briefly, meditation can be seen as the discipline of quietening the mind using various forms of mental exercises (such as repeating a word/phrase or 'mantra') – the results of which may be to bring us into a deep awareness of the present moment and/or expanded awareness of Ultimate Reality or God, depending on the person's spiritual beliefs. Contemplation is usually concerned with holding the attention upon thoughts or images of the divine in order to draw closer to God. Prayer usually suggests an inner dialogue, entreaty or request of God/the Absolute. These are very short definitions for the purposes of this discussion; in practice, meditation, prayer and contemplation are terms often used interchangeably, and the practices overlap. Definitions thereby become rather meaningless – one might meditate before praying or enter a state of expanded awareness after a period of contemplation. A friend of mine who is a Greek Orthodox monk believes that trying to define them is rather pointless: 'In the end,' he said to me recently, 'Whether you chat to God or mantra your way to stillness, it's all much of a muchness. Really all you are being asked to do is just shut up and listen!' A Buddhist nun known to me said she would meditate on it when I asked her what the difference was. Ten years later, she is still meditating on it.

The Latin root of the word 'meditation' (*mederi*) means to heal. Much research shows the positive health benefits to practitioners of meditation, such as greater intimacy with and reduced fear of other people, increased energy, greater relaxation, less susceptibility to depression, greater awareness of good diet, exercise and posture, and less use of smoking, drinking and drugs. There also appear to be benefits for psychological stability, lower anxiety, lower rates of breathing, pulse and blood pressure, improved internal locus of control and a sense of being effective in the world rather than a victim of circumstance (for summaries of the many studies, see Kabat-Zinn, 1996; Woodham & Peters, 1997; Santorelli, 1999; Graham, 1999; Segal et al., 2002).

While much work has been done, and doctors like Jon Kabat-Zinn and others have been at the cutting edge of integrating meditation into mainstream health care, there is still a long way to travel. For example, of the 63,914 research projects registered with the National Research Register, only six are associated with the effects of yoga/meditation (National Research Register, 2002). Most carers within orthodox health care still see it very much as fringe activity, despite the proven benefits. And the benefits are two-fold. It's not just about the direct impact of meditation upon the wellbeing of the individual practitioner, but also about the way the benefits spill over (if they are working as carers) into therapeutic relationships with clients. It makes us better able to 'be with' people, to remain 'clear-eyed' and still, and within the storm of the illness experience.

SANCTUARY

Sometimes work can feel like we are stuck in stagnant and marshy waters, the endless toil broken by the prospect of the next holiday as a chance for respite. Caught up in the grand drama of caring, sometimes the only sanctuary would seem to be to fly free of it, if only for a little while.

Sanctuary – the idea of a safe sacred place where we are free from the pursuit by others, a place to re-member and re-collect who we are in the midst of all this 'stuff', this 'stuff' being our work in the swamp of human suffering. Many health-care staff take sanctuary by literally flying away from it – but after a holiday we may come back to the way things always were. The temporary refreshment soon wears off as we hit the pile of work awaiting us. Nothing has really changed. Meanwhile, many studies have shown (see Chapters 1 and 2) that we can find other ways of escaping from the pressures of caring – not all of them positive, such as increased likelihood to resort to drink, drugs, smoking, serial relationships, suicide and more. Snow and Willard's (1989) study, for example, suggested that up to 80 per cent of nurses may be really struggling in their roles and seek to drown this struggle in a wide range of damaging behaviours like these.

Finding the time and place to re-collect ourselves is important; otherwise we can continue to feel dismembered by the conflicting demands at work and home, pulled this way and that as we seek to meet the needs of others. This is all made worse by the often-inhospitable managerial cultures and dis-spiriting environments in which we work (see Chapter 2).

Most of our hospital buildings, clinics and other workplaces are clinically clean yet spiritually dead. They are built to be functional, but without the concept of sacred architecture, where buildings are pleasing to the eye and bring added healing benefits from their precise proportions and perspectives (Mann, 1993). Interestingly, Florence Nightingale held great store by this in her pioneering design for hospitals – a notion now long dead, it seems, in the minds of most modern architects and hospital planners, who sacrifice the wholesomeness (holiness) of a building on the altar of efficiency. This economy may be a false one; the dispiriting environment may in the long term simply add to staff and patient sickness. Some settings, such as the Glasgow Homeopathic Hospital (Wright, 2004b) and the leading-edge Planetree Hospital in California, are setting examples of best practice in creating truly holistic environments, but as yet such places are still relatively rare in mainstream health systems.

A demolition job on much of our health service infrastructure is not possible, but we can take some steps to mitigate their worst effects and restore a sense of the sacred space of healing work (the very essence of the original concept of the hospital). We can look again at that dusty old hospital chapel and reinvigorate it perhaps as a multi-faith sanctuary for meditation and contemplation, or create sacred spaces elsewhere on site where there is space for stillness and silence. This can obviously be difficult in settings where space is at a premium, but it can be done with a bit of imagination.

I know of one colleague who has created a small shrine area in one corner of his office – a place filled with symbols of spiritual significance to him. McMann (1998) gives some beautiful examples of how this can be done without being intrusive. My colleague's office has become the place where everyone seems to go in search of peace and solace – despite some initial scepticism and funny looks.

Gordon (1998) has argued that sanctuaries for finding stillness and solitude should be built in the workplace, especially as we live in a largely non-secular society. Meanwhile, pupils at Stocktonwood Junior and Infant School in one of the most deprived areas of Liverpool have created a 'quiet place' – a room offering peace, calm and support from a counsellor. The quiet place on the campus at the University of York is a sanctuary centred on an old Georgian gazebo. At the Sacred Space Foundation we have worked with several NHS settings to develop 'caring for the carers' practices, which embrace the idea of setting up a sanctuary in the workplace. Our retreat centres, like many other places of retreat, have purpose-built sanctuaries for silence and meditation. Victoria Stone (2000) provides one example of how many people are now bringing a sense of the sacred into the healthcare environment – not least with the creation with Agnes Bourne of a labyrinth and sanctuary at the California Pacific Medical Center. She and professionals like her are showing how the clinical and the spiritual do not have to be in opposition but can indeed be in harmony.

It's one thing to have a quiet place to retreat to when we feel stressed at work or just in need of a quiet moment to ourselves. (It should be possible for all staff at work to do this and much more healthy than a desperate smoke outside the main entrance!) It's another, however, to be able to make best use of it. This needs two things. The first is an organisational culture that accepts and gives permission for staff to take sanctuary for a short time. Second, we often need preparation ourselves (such as a meditation training programme) to be able to make best use of it. The most important sanctuary we have is within ourselves, but sitting quietly with that can be difficult at first and downright scary for some.

Coming home to the still, quiet space within ourselves is arrival at sanctuary. From this safe, sacred space we are far better equipped to deal with the buffeting of our everyday lives. Shifting the environment helps, but this is only a gateway to a shift in our thinking about how we best take care of ourselves and the real source of our strength in our work.

JUST SITTING

If meditation has much to commend it, as suggested above, it does not come entirely without risk. And while the health benefits are laudable, it has to be remembered from a spiritual perspective that meditation down the years has been taught for quite different reasons. Indeed it could be argued that the health gains are mere side effects to the real intent of meditation to approach God, the Absolute, the deepest Self, depending on your perspective. Who wouldn't want to buy a product that offers so much yet demands so little – all you need is a bit of time, no drugs, no special equipment. As a meditation teacher I am often asked to guide people into it to help them cope with stress – and it can be an impressive quick fix. But there is more to it than seeking another emotional condom to cope with the realities of modern life. Indeed to suggest that we can meditate with a purpose is a spiritual oxymoron as I observed earlier, for the goal of meditation, paradoxically, is to be goal-less.

When we meditate, we learn to sit — that is, not just to still ourselves physically but also to get our minds to sit still as well. Try it now as you read this — just put the book down and close your eyes for a minute or two. What happens? Chances are, if you are not an experienced meditator, all you will get is what the Buddhists call 'monkey mind' — anything but stillness as your mind leaps from one thing to the next and gets caught up by internal and external distractions. And that's just for starters. Not by accident have meditation traditions throughout history — from the first Hindu gurus or the Desert Fathers of early Christianity to modern-day reputable teachers such as Jack Kornfield or Larry Le Shan — emphasised caution.

Meditation, the quietening of the mind, is not just about seeking health benefits, indeed it could be argued that these are mere spin-offs from the deeper reasons for meditation. As we learn to sit (and it has to be learned, there are no short cuts, no easy answers — it takes discipline) we may be transported beyond ordinary perceptions of self and reality that cannot easily be put into words.

> *There remains no part of one's being that is hungry. There is a feeling of everlasting satisfaction in knowing something that the knower can never put into words. It is the knowledge that mystics call self-realization, and that is recognized by some religious-minded people as God consciousness, and by philosophical minds as cosmic consciousness.*
> Inayat Khan, cited in Witteveen, 1997

Meditation is therefore not just about health goals, though these are laudable benefits. And we could construct a very good evidence-based case for using meditation far more than we do in our health services. What illness is not associated with stress?

Meditation can take many forms and comes from a rich history of the desire of human beings to achieve a deeper connection with the divine, with the cosmos. It is not without risks and should not be undertaken lightly, or without proper teaching, supervision and ongoing support (I am therefore deeply sceptical of the benefits, indeed safety, of 'off-the-shelf' meditation packages found in any bookstore). Meditation can be blissful and exhilarating but it can also be distressing and subversive; as we explore the 'interior castle', as St Theresa of Avila described it, our vision of who we are and why we are here can be challenged. It can expose us to all manner of internal shadows and difficulties that may have been long buried in our psyche. There is a great renewal of meditation taking place in the Christian Church, influenced not least by the leading work of the Benedictine monk John Main (1988). Meditation may not only be personally subversive, but also organisationally. After all, if our connection with 'all that is' can be unmediated by religious hierarchies, then will they still be needed?

THE SILENT MIRROR

Sitting in silence can be one of the most difficult, even terrifying, things we can experience and often we will do almost anything to avoid it. A dear friend of mine is a lay preacher in the Church of England and she has sought to gradually introduce more contemplative silence into her services. I think she got as far as six minutes before the parishioners began to complain that 'It went on a bit too long.'

Why should it be so uncomfortable, even scary? In stillness and silence we may witness all the bits of ourselves we would rather not look at, or the triviality of so much of our lives that we kid ourselves is really important. In silence we may hear what we would rather not hear – the inner voice that calls us 'home', threatening all that we have come to believe ourselves to be. Steve Smith (cited in Holdom, 1999), the round-the-world sailor, wrote of the effect of being alone and silent at sea:

> *Your brain is crying out for something to think about. You go through every little thing you thought of. Then all your history is gone. Then you go through all your future plans, drawings, designs. Nothing is happening, so there's nothing to talk about there. Then you're stuck and that's when the panic sets in and there's no panic greater than not having anything to think about. It's really quite frightening and that's when people start to go insane and dream of mermaids.*

Our minds will deploy every trick in the book to avoid the effects of silence, because unconsciously, if not consciously, we know not only what a frightening place it can be, but also that what lies beyond it, beyond Smith's fear of madness, is the possibility that something more than our egos exists – the possibility of which would threaten the ego's belief that it is in charge. Our egos do not like to be sussed out for the finite ephemera they are.

Bede Griffiths tells of the complaints of monks at Downside, where he taught meditation:'I feel I am wasting my time,' they would often say.'I sit there and nothing happens and my mind wanders about. I ought to be doing something'. (Griffiths, cited in Wakeman, 2002). In his splendid poem *The Four Quartets*, Eliot (1944) writes of that point in silence of 'the growing terror of nothing to think about'. Doing or thinking about something, anything, anything at all, becomes preferable to facing silence. Writing of the contemporary technological lifestyle, the Islamic scholar, Dr Sayyed Hossein Nasr says how we extend distraction into the material world, especially full nowadays with the seductions of electronic gadgetry, which can 'cause an eclipse of the spiritual life, of contemplation, of tranquillity, and of more profound communication' and lead to 'an agitated soul that jumps from moment to moment, event to event, and does not want to rest upon itself, does not want to contemplate' (cited in Roemischer, 2003).

So, the restless mind has innumerable tricks to keep us from stillness and silence, where we can feel so unsafe. Paradoxically, when we get past the stream of consciousness and overcome our fears, it is here that we may discover the deeper truth of our true nature, our soul, that which the Quakers describe as 'That of God in everyone' (Pym, 1999). Pym cites John Southall, a nineteenth-century Quaker printer who wrote of his first experience of sitting in silence, as is the custom at Quaker meetings for worship, where the 'pandemonium of voices reaching my ears, a thousand clamouring notes from within' gave way to a profound stillness wherein he began to hear a 'still small voice in the depths of my being that began to speak with an inexpressible tenderness, power and comfort.' Throughout the ages, religious and spiritual traditions across the globe have used techniques of prayer, meditation and contemplation to transcend the experience of ordinary reality and the cacophony of siren voices in our minds and to reach deeper levels of experience and knowledge about the nature of the true Self, of Ultimate Reality. For some this may simply be coming to rest in the loving nature of their humanity, to others a realisation of the universal consciousness, to yet others the connection to God. While the traditions and beliefs emphasise different approaches and perspectives on what can or should happen, the endpoint is fairly consistent – a transformation of who we are in the world through the quietening of the mind.

When we do not give time to silence and stillness, we put off such discoveries, and push our minds and bodies to ever-greater limits – resulting in all manner of health problems, stress and burnout. On all counts, people who commit to some form of spiritual path, including practices encouraging stillness and silence, tend to be healthier and longer lived and able to cope better with the strains and stresses of ordinary life, as suggested above. At work, most of us who work in health care can find ourselves in slightly controlled (and sometimes not so controlled) manic hospitals and clinics. For most it's like living in a vast episode of Monty Python or Eastenders – depending on how you experience it – either somewhat crazy and surreal or full of over-the-top dramas and turmoil. There seems to be neither time nor place to re-mind ourselves that we are more than the roles we adopt, and so we get caught in the act, except there's no one there to press the button to interrupt the episode with the advertising break. We end up in some long unbroken drama, like actors on the stage, and like actors we tend to burn out when we are stuck in the role or forget what is real – the role I play or the real 'me'.

Thus to, literally, re-mind ourselves we need two immediate provisions – the first is the space for silence, stillness and solitude (sanctuary, as discussed above); the second is the ability to make best use of it and not have it drive us even more crazy. A few enlightened places I have worked in have set about creating quiet sanctuaries for staff and offered access to meditation or contemplation programmes so that the silence can be used well, with the necessary tools to enter it safely and comfortably. But such places are as yet few and far between. I would argue that such places are essential for staff wellbeing, despite the pressures on accommodation or other priorities. While many places have hospital chapels, for example, smaller workplaces do not. And even the chapel can be a busy place, or there may be patients present when it is from patients and other carers that the staff member needs to escape, even for a little while.

There is a story told of Carl Jung and one of his students. The great philosopher-psychologist told the student to go into a room, lock the door, and stay there silent for two hours. After half an hour the student emerged unable to stand it any longer and Jung said, 'If you can't spend two hours with yourself, how do you expect anybody else to spend all day with you?'

He had a point, perhaps. And, remember, a growing body of evidence, as I have touched on in previous chapters, points to the wellbeing of patients being improved when they are in the hands of carers and in environments where the staff feel OK about themselves too. I remember my time as a student nurse with dear Sister Calvert; she ran her orthopaedic ward with firm compassion – and one thing she was firm about was the rest hour in the afternoon. Nothing and nobody, barring emergencies, was allowed to disturb that quiet time, which she saw as essential to the patients' recovery. I remember Pat, a district nurse, who would always find five minutes in the day to stop by the park en route and sit silently in her car, looking at the trees to, as she put it, 'restore my soul'. Does your schedule, workplace or home have time and space for the sanctuary and healing power of silence?

AND ON THE SEVENTH DAY . . .

Thomas Merton (cited in Muller, 1999) posits that:

> There is a pervasive form of contemporary violence . . . [and that is] activism and overwork. The rush and pressure of modern life are a form, perhaps the most common form, of its innate violence. To allow oneself to be carried away by a multitude of conflicting concerns, to surrender to too many demands, to commit oneself to too many projects, to want to help everyone in everything, is to succumb to violence. The frenzy of our activism neutralises our work for peace. It destroys our own inner capacity for peace. It destroys the fruitfulness of our own work, because it kills the root of our inner wisdom which makes it fruitful.

We all need rites to reinforce what it is to be human, and one of these rites is the regular sanctuary of solitude, silence and stillness. Contemporary life makes little space as I have suggested – driven by the imperative to be economically productive and the scariness that stillness can bring. When we are not being busy, we may be confronted by a kind of spiritual agoraphobia – a fear of the open space within ourselves.

Healthcare practitioners of all sorts, as we have seen in Chapter 2, are particularly vulnerable to the violence of 'busyness' and to getting caught up in the co-dependence of constant activity. Of course, we rationalise this through our commitment to our work, the 'calling' or commitment of our occupation and the deeply rooted belief that we must be constantly giving of ourselves in the face of infinite demand from patients and a 'system' that never provides us with enough resources to do our work. Many health settings are indeed tough places to work in, in terms of the work to be done and the ability to meet it, but other factors are also present.

The merry-go-round of opportunity for endless activity provides us with fertile soil to plant the seeds of our own workaholism, keeping busy dealing with the outer stuff so that we don't have to confront the inner stuff – the sources of our interior weariness and uncertainty. And, make no mistake about it, we all suffer to some degree from this inner/outer struggle, and there are only two kinds of people we can identify as a result – those who are honest and aware of this and those in denial!

The Keep Sunday Special campaign in the UK, in the face of an enormous cultural shift away from worship at the altar of the church (towards the altar of consumption in the supermarket), has a point. Regardless of the underpinning religious beliefs or otherwise of the campaign, there is a thread of concern here that our culture of busyness seduces us away from the possibilities of stillness. Even the all-powerful God of the Old Testament had to take a break on day seven! Libertarian, capitalist values of freedom of choice are beguiling – assuming that those who wish to take a Sabbath rest can do so and those who don't can shop. Such freedoms may in fact be enslaving without the social and personal backdrop of rituals and conventions that encourage and legitimise rest.

Many are now questioning the consequences of creating a society where one day rolls onward into the next with no distinctive pattern for rest and recuperation. Muller (1999), for example, reminds us of the significance of rebuilding the idea of the Sabbath in our lives, not just from a religious perspective, but in order to have space and time committed to rest, renewal, reflection, relationship and recuperation. To fully express our human spirit we need to be busy, but we need stillness too. This can be hugely difficult to achieve where so many external and internal signals call us to keep active.

The restoration of a sabbatical, in the broadest sense of the word, might do much to aid our passage through the fraught world of nursing work. I know of groups of nurses who have introduced quiet sanctuaries in the workplace where staff can take time out, even if only for a few minutes in the day. Others, like me, practise meditation or t'ai chi daily. A Muslim friend stops five times a day to pray, a Buddhist neighbour meditates for an hour each morning and evening. Integration into our normal daily lives is the key. In the world of the spiritual supermarket, there are thousands of options to choose from. Getting rid of the television was also an interesting choice in my case. Apart from a brief sense of social exclusion when you could not discuss with friends the latest escapades of *Big Brother*, this quickly passed into a recognition of how much richer life became with other things, not least a greater opportunity to do nothing. After a while it was possible to bring the TV back, but to its rightful place as an occasional resource for learning and entertainment and not the regular backdrop it had become, as in so many homes.

Jack Kornfield (2000) writes:

> *A spirit of service to one another and to ourselves grows . . . out of moments of remembering, moments of prayer and blessing . . . To beat for our whole life, the heart must restore itself in the stillness before each new beat. Spiritual maturity also requires such periods of Sabbath, where we step out of commercial time into that which is timeless.*

There is strength in the argument for restoring Sabbath time into our daily working lives and for regular days, perhaps each week, to spend less time doing and more time being. It doesn't have to be a Sunday for an individual Sabbath time: the idea of having a sacred space of time in the week for ourselves could be adjusted to suit individual need. I have one friend who finds it convenient to keep Mondays as her Sabbath. Some would hold that a traditional Sunday is important, but other faiths would have different views. Whatever the view, the important matter seems to be that both individually and collectively there seems to be a strong case for a restful day in the week that is not dedicated to the outer life, but the inner.

THE INNER SANCTUM

It is worth remembering that people who are 'present' reside in their own inner sanctuary. Sanctuary is wherever we are. It transcends the need, when we are in this way of being, for a special time or place. Illness is a 'day-by-day, minute-by-minute attack upon the soul' (Gordon, 1997). The suffering that emerges from such an assault upon the very core of our being can be relieved in the respite we find in a clear-eyed carer. No matter how brief the contact, our presence can be a form of sanctuary as well. Consider the words of that great philosopher, Winnie the Pooh (Milne, 1982):

> *Piglet sidled up to Pooh from behind.*
> *'Pooh' he whispered.*
> *'Yes Piglet?'*
> *'Nothing' said Piglet, taking Pooh's paw. 'I just wanted to be sure of you.'*

We feel better when we are sure of people and we care better when we are sure of ourselves. Attentive, still and resting, the very essence of meditation, the work gets done as we stay in the moment. Meditation is healing and healing is meditation. Being in the moment, we become sanctuary for those in need by our very mindful, attentive and aware presence. Like my mum – just making the socks better.

CHAPTER 9

PEEPING THROUGH THE CRACK IN THE DOORS OF PERCEPTION — REFLECTIONS ON THE PERILS AND PITFALLS OF THE QUICK WAYS TO GOD

We had the experience but missed the meaning . . .

TS Eliot, 1944

I REMEMBER THE 60S

The fly agaric (*Amanita muscaria*), the bright red toadstool with the white spots, grows wild in the fields around my home. Its imagery is found in countless illustrations of legends and fairy tales, finding its way even to the red and white garb of Father Christmas, whose shamanic origins predate Christianity by many millennia. Regarded as poisonous, it is also hallucinogenic and believed to be the source of the legendary 'soma', the food of the gods, the inspiration for many early religious writings such as the Indian Rig Veda (Jesse, 2002). Plants and fungi like this have, in the hands of priests and shamans, traditionally provided the bridge to what Aldous Huxley (an ardent user of hallucinogens himself) called the 'doors of perception' (Huxley, 1954). In some parts of the world, they still (legally) form part of religious ceremonies, such as peyote in the Navaho 'church' in the USA. A Huichol shaman (cited in Schultes & Hofmann, 1992) from Central America honours the buds of the peyote cactus, the ingestion of which produces effects that are of profound significance to the religiosity of his whole culture: 'Speak to the Peyote with your heart, with your thoughts. And the Peyote sees your heart. And if you have luck, you will hear things and receive things that are invisible to others, but that God has given you to pursue your path.'

Rastafarians in the UK have faced a running battle with the authorities for the legalisation of marijuana because of its traditional use in their religious practices. The use of ayahuasca has spread widely in Brazil beyond the original boundaries of aboriginal rites into the Christian Church. If meditation (and its close allies prayer and contemplation), as suggested in Chapter 8, are probably the most widespread form of spiritual practice, common to many religions and spiritual paths, the same must apply to the use of a wide range of substances used to connect ultimately to reality, however we chose to perceive it.

Synthesised substances like LSD or MDMA (ecstasy) and many others are readily available nowadays despite the best efforts of prohibition. Indeed it was only with the rise of the counterculture in the 1960s that we saw such substances banned. Drugs that had once been available to an elite had become mass-produced, and to have the masses following Timothy Leary's famous call (Badiner & Hunt, 2002) to 'turn on, tune in, drop out' was more than much of society could bear.

What was it they said about the 1960s – 'If you can remember them, you weren't there'? I remember them, though these were my teenage years when like millions of my compatriots I grew my hair long, quit the nine to five and spent some time travelling abroad before falling back into convention (at least outwardly) by getting a job in the NHS when I returned. Unlike Bill Clinton, who famously did not inhale, I did try cannabis when I moved to swinging London in 1967 (but couldn't and never have been able to smoke, so after an embarrassing half an hour of spluttering and choking, I gave up the effort and stuck with beer). Later at a student party I was offered mescaline and after a four-hour, deep and meaningful relationship with the sound of my finger on a windowpane, I took up watching paint dry instead as a more exciting pastime. My aversion or inability to get into mind-altering substances did have one pay-off for all my friends; I could always be relied upon to get them home in one piece or their heads out of the toilet.

A GLIMPSE IS NOT ENLIGHTENMENT

Psychoactive drugs have been divided into four groups (Schultes & Hofmann, 1992) – the analgesics and euphorics (opium, coca), sedatives and tranquillisers (reserpine), hypnotics (kava-kava), and hallucinogens or psychotomimetics (peyote, marijuana).

> *Most of these groups modify only the mood, either stimulating or calming it. But the last group produces deep changes in the sphere of experience, in perception of reality, even space and time and in consciousness itself. Depersonalisation may occur. Without loss of consciousness, the subject enters a dream world, which often appears more real than the normal world. Colours are frequently experienced in indescribable brilliance; objects may*

lose their symbolic character, standing detached and assuming increased significance since they seem to possess their own existence. The psychic changes and abnormal consciousness induced by hallucinogens are so far removed from similarity with ordinary life that it is impossible to describe them in the language of daily living. A person under the effects of an hallucinogen forsakes his familiar world and operates under other standards, in strange dimensions and in different time.

Schultes and Hofmann, 1992

What Schultes and Hofmann have named as abnormal reality is termed 'non-ordinary' reality by Grof, who has used a technique called 'holotropic breath-work' to induce similar states of consciousness without the aid of ingested substances. Grof (1980) sought to induce a condition of non-ordinary reality in his patients and students when LSD became illegal in the USA. There is a striking similarity in the words used by Schultes and Hofmann to those used to describe the pattern of the mystical experience. Underhill's (1993) classic text on mysticism, more importantly the descriptions of the mystical state by mystics themselves, bears many of the hallmarks of the hallucinogenic experience, of a state of non-ordinary reality. The mystic frequently reports passing beyond an ordinary consciousness to experience the world and the cosmos differently and to ultimately achieve union with the divine. The spoken or written word is often seen as too restrictive a means to express what the mystic experiences in a state of non-ordinary reality. Only when words are stretched in poetry or stream-of-consciousness prose and other forms of art such as film, music and painting has it been possible to come close to expressing what it is like.

Societies across the globe have sought to prohibit the use of hallucinogens. People who see things differently tend to want to question the status quo and change things – not something to which the political establishment is always responsive. The risks to the health of users are often cited as reasons for restriction. Many of these substances are indeed dangerous if used carelessly, but the extremity of the sanctions used seems to be out of proportion and far more heavy-handed than the actual health risks demand. Pinchbeck (2003) notes how the psychedelic/hallucinogen movement of the 1960s came to be seen as a direct threat to the social order when he reports how these substances could be used as 'deconditioning and deprogramming agents' to 'break the trance of the consensus culture'. They were a key element in the revolutionary movements that swept across many parts of the globe in the late 1960s, and many elements of Western culture at the time reeled with alarm at the prospect.

Likewise, religions have not always looked kindly on mystics for related but different reasons. The mystic, after all, requires no priest or religious officiate to mediate between themselves and the divine. The mystic has direct access, communion and union with the Divine, Ultimate Reality, the Absolute. They enter a state of non-ordinary reality at will or involuntarily (Underhill, 1993) and do so without the aid of any psychoactive substances. The mystic, despite the fact that almost all the great faiths are founded on the mystical experience of their earliest exponents, represents as much a threat to orthodoxy in religion as the drug user does to social and political order. Consequently both groups have found themselves looked upon with varying degrees of suspicion, not to say hostility, at various times in history.

There are differences, however. The person using hallucinogens may do so for many motives, including the desire to reach a transcendent state and connect with the Absolute, but may just as easily seek it to drop out of the challenges of living in ordinary reality for a while, or simply be seeking fun. Some mystics may have occasionally reported the use of drugs to break through their initial barriers to connection, but tend to eschew them in favour of the spiritual practice of mystical awakening without the rocket fuel of mind-altering substances.

CONTEXT AND INTENTION

Thus people have been trying for millennia to get to God (arguably success-fully) using what in modern usage have become known as the 'entheogens' – substances that induce an altered state of consciousness associated with an experience of the divine. The term 'entheogen' (from the Greek for '*God with-in*') was first used by Ruck and his colleagues for a class of psychoactives that had become debased, in their view, because of their associations with pop and revolutionary culture (Jesse, 2002).

Many drugs now readily available to us, from the legal (alcohol, caffeine, tobacco) to the illegal (cocaine, cannabis, mescaline), were once used by initi-ated individuals, rarely and sparingly, in tribal cultures. They were not the stuff of mass consumption. Tobacco, for example, once used sparingly, was con-sidered a drug of great spiritual power. Aboriginal peoples elevated these substances beyond other medicines, which only had physical effects on the body in treating diseases. These plant extracts that induced altered states became sacred, the holy of holies for what they offered, and they were therefore reserved for special times, people and places. Casual use was prohibited as it was seen to diminish the spiritual potential and original intent. A Native American once told me, 'A white man goes into his church and talks *about* Jesus, an Indian goes into his tepee and talks *to* Jesus.'

Modern synthesised substances such as LSD and ecstasy, which are illegal, have nevertheless spread widely in our culture and are readily and easily avail-able to those who know where to look. The genie is out of the bottle, and despite the best international efforts, regulation and massive investment both in financial and manpower terms, these substances have spread to all parts of the world. The original entheogens and their modern counterparts are consumed on a massive scale for leisure and pleasure. What were once sacred substances with rare and profound uses have been proletarianised, commodified like any other marketable object. Some would argue that this has dumbed down their original intent and made available to the masses, often quite cheaply, agents of conscious change – some of which can be downright dangerous when not used carefully. Others might argue that, at last, access to the numinous is (more) available to all and might be of service in the world to wake us all up to a deeper reality so that we might appreciate and take care of the present one better than we do currently.

The context matters too. Taking ecstasy at a wild party, laced with alcohol, boosted by amphetamines and driven by rap, will have a hugely different impact (as some of the arrivals in any accident and emergency department amply demonstrate) than ingestion after fasting and ritual preparation, inclusion in a sacred ceremony and environment, and guidance by a spiritual master. I have known people take ecstasy at a party, have a wild time dancing and then enjoy hyper-passionate sex afterwards, and simply see it as a great night out. I have known others spend days without food, hours in prayer and contemplation and reading sacred texts, and be guided through the process by their priest or mentor, and have what they believe is a direct experience of God. However, even with the best intentional preparation to reach out to the divine, as Christine Longaker has pointed out, we can have glimpses of enlightenment through various spiritual practices, brief mystical insights or drug-induced altered states of consciousness, but a glimpse of enlightenment is not enlightenment itself (Longaker, 1998). A mystical experience may be mimicked, but there seems to be no way of bypassing the long term hard discipline of spiritual practice even if there has been an initial opening of the doors of perception. There are no short cuts around the emotional work and the spiritual labour if we are ever to approach healthily, for ourselves and others, the true essence of our being.

It has been noted that even if the ego-crushing effect of the entheogens obtains, there is no certainty as to what might take its place without safe and tried and tested means of support. LSD and its proponents, like Leary for example, 'cannot provide the answers to the most profound issue exposed by the LSD trip: once the individual ego was liberated from its social role, from the well-worn grooves of Western society's game machinery, what was it supposed to do?' (Pinchbeck, 2003). It seems that regardless of the hallucinogen used, one effect is to lay open to the mind the possibility that all that it had held dear as certainty may not be so. As we step through the doors of perception, ordinary life and our place in it may never quite be the same again.

However, this is by no means certain. The drug-induced experience may leave the user wanting more (to repeat it), or failing to trust it simply because it was under chemical influence and therefore not 'real', or letting it fade into the dusty and unused filing cabinets of memory. The mystic too can have this hunger for repetition, and this is made part of the mystic's spiritual practice as they learn that even the desire for the numinous must ultimately be surrendered in order for connection to Source to return and deepen.

It may be that the entheogens mimic the spontaneous or induced (through non-chemical spiritual practices such as meditation) spiritual awakenings of the mystic, but there are attendant risks of reliance upon them. How and why they work is still not yet fully understood. It may be that the mystic intuitively and intentionally taps into that part of the brain that may be 'wired for God' (Newberg et al., 2001) while the entheogen user is getting a similar effect by a chemical interaction in the same place.

Pinchbeck's own reliance upon hallucinogens for his shamanic spiritual awakening, and his belief in the continued use of them to stay awakened, further illustrates one of the traps of this approach. Without the inner work to ground and integrate the glimpses, they require continued use to stay 'there'. (It is worth noting that, in the case of shamanism, the groundbreaking work of reintroducing this spiritual practice into cultures where it has died out has been achievable without drugs by the likes of leaders in the field such as Michael Harner. Shamans are often associated with drug use, but this is not a universal or continuous phenomenon.)

A GLIMPSE, BUT WHAT THEN?

The trick, if there is one, is to expand and integrate the mystical experience, however it is induced. As Walsh argues:

> For those people who are graced with mystical experience – whether induced spontaneously, contemplatively or chemically – the crucial question is what to do with it. It can be allowed to fade; it can be ignored or even dismissed, or perhaps clung to as a psychological or spiritual trophy. Or it can be consciously used as a source of inspiration and guidance to direct one's life along more beneficial directions. One such direction – indeed the one recommended by the great mystics – is to undertake the necessary contemplative training of life and mind so as to be able to re-enter and expand the mystical state. The aim is to extend a single peak experience to a recurring plateau experience, to change an altered state into an altered trait.
>
> Walsh, 2002

Integration, if we are willing to do the work leads us beyond the need for hallucinogens and glimpses and flashes of illumination and enlightenment then become an 'abiding light' (Smith, 1964).

Our culture's ambivalent attitude towards drugs has limited a meaningful dialogue about them, especially how they could be effectively used in health care. It may be that the entheogens have a rightful place in modern health care for short-term and specific use. Many people currently clogging the beds of our psychiatric units, for example, are in fact in spiritual crisis, a crisis of meaning and purpose in their lives and the cracking of their personhood as some deep wound bursts open. Western psychiatry, in thrall to reductionist biological models of mental illness and worshipping at the altars of multi-national drug companies, has got itself trapped up a blind alley, whereas controlled access to entheogens and the wider use of spiritual counselling and therapeutic communities could offer better ways out. If the entheogens can awaken people, under careful guidance, to a deeper reality then they may offer a source of healing for many contemporary problems.

Psychiatrists and psychotherapists have become the new priest-shamans. Unfortunately, the legally available drugs and techniques of choice serve largely to batten down the hatches rather than open people up (safely) to what their souls are crying out to be. Our culture is going to have to take some brave and radical steps if the entheogens are to find their therapeutic use realised, and reclaim them from the recreational black market.

Meanwhile the fly agarics in my garden will burst forth as usual to be nibbled away by mice and voles. Heaven only knows what they are seeing!

CHAPTER 10

OF GODS AND GURUS – FEAR AND LOATHING IN THE SPIRITUAL QUEST

For pray do not . . . spin your airy fables about noon or sun or the other objects in the sky and in the universe so far removed from us and so varied in their natures, until you have scrutinised and come to know yourselves. After that, we may perhaps believe you when you hold forth on other subjects; but before you establish who you yourselves are, do not think that you will ever become capable of acting as judges or trustworthy witnesses in other matters.

Philo (Jewish philosopher and mystic, late first-century BC)

HOW DOES HE TREAT HIS WIFE?

He was not a particularly big man, but what he lacked in stature he made up for in swagger. His wife had accompanied him to the conference, to be seen most of the time dutifully following him, always a pace or two behind wherever he went. His lecture, delivered with studied fervour and evangelical zeal, had much of the audience either loving or hating him, depending less on content than how you were able to receive the style of delivery. Perhaps more informative amidst the peroration from the wise man, the expert, the spiritual guru who had been invited to address us about the meaning of life, was a telling moment. It was one of those flickers in the stream of events that suddenly shifts your perception of things, which although the occurrence may seem minor, takes on greater import and changes everything else as a consequence. A larger matter was at stake – the lecture was in full flow and seemingly great truths were on offer as the audience, or at least most of it, hung on his every word as if at any moment we might grasp the great truth that would lead us to enlightenment. His confidence and passion poured out to us, he spoke like a man who 'knew'. He spoke like a man used to being listened to.

Then it happened, unnoticed by most. It may have been a momentary lapse (perhaps I took it out of proportion), but the effect was as if there had been a sudden awakening from a dream. In the midst of a session that should have been about a path to the divine (which, it was assumed, because of his CV and his presence here, he had already trod), there was a revealing distraction. A problem arose with the audio–visual aids he had brought with him – a number of slides and overheads. His face instantly contorted with anger and he snapped at his wife, who was operating the equipment. She, mouse-like, took the blame, sorted things out and the lecture on love and compassion proceeded. I lost my attention, already wavering because of his 'in-your-face' style of presentation, on anything he had to say thereafter. What was being presented as truth now just seemed like a big lie, a falsity, 'fur coat and no knickers' as my mother used to say – a front dressed up for appearances, but beneath the veneer nothing of substance. It was a pretence: high ideals ungrounded in reality.

It only lasted a moment and could have been interpreted in various ways. But that fraction of a second's display allowed some words of Larry Le Shan (1974) to surface for me, that I had read recently. I heard the man's lecture from what seemed like a great distance after that, and in my mind's eye, like a neon sign over the stage, I could see emblazoned Larry's questioning words: 'How does he treat his wife?' In other words, we can check if someone is authentic by looking at the way they conduct their lives. If they talk of peace and love, for example, are they practising it not just in their fight for social justice but, in their conduct with their nearest and dearest?

THE GURU

In this age of the spiritual supermarket, more people than ever have abandoned orthodoxy and authority figures in their search for health and spirituality. Indeed, as some studies have suggested, much of the search for health in the complementary therapies movement is often linked to a spiritual search as well (Thorsons, 1999). Gurus, and those who see themselves as such, appear to be on every street corner, advertising in every New Age journal (and not so New Age) or popping up in TV programmes. But the term 'guru' appears to have been debased, at least in Western culture where the word is now sloppily applied to almost any expert or pundit in their field. In the East, where the term arose, it refers quite specifically to people who have undertaken considerable spiritual practice to come to a realised state, a level of consciousness that holds but also transcends ordinary reality. They have achieved what is known by various names as enlightenment, diamond consciousness, sky of mind, divine union – the authority that comes with their wisdom, knowledge and direct experience. The guru does not just talk about it, they embody it.

Mariana Caplan (2002), in her excellent dissection of the guru principle, refers specifically to their role in relation to spirituality. To use the term in relation to any other occupation is to dumb down what is a profound concept and to belittle the significance that the guru has with the follower. She writes of two types of authority:

> *Relative authorities include those who, human like the rest of us but perhaps one or many steps ahead along the path, function as mentors or guides; absolute authorities include the gurus and masters – whatever we call them – who are seen either as incarnations of the divine, or as powerful (if not flawless) vehicles of transmission for divine direction.*

Ram Dass (1997) suggests quite simply, 'A teacher points the way, a guru *is* the way.' The guru teaches like the teacher, but has gone further – the guru not only 'knows' but has integrated this knowing fully into their way of being in the world. A teacher may talk of love and compassion; a guru *is* love and compassion. Gurus are the practitioners of what they preach. They have paid their dues, having done perhaps many decades of spiritual practice (and invariably continuing to do so) and now make themselves, humbly, in the service of others so that they too may come to 'know'.

THE LIFESTYLE GURU – EGO TOAST FOR BREAKFAST

Much of the New Age approach to the spiritual is about making ourselves feel better. I know of no authentic spiritual path that might not actually make you feel a good deal worse at times. For if spiritual practice is anything it is about subverting the desires and power of the ego, our personhoods, the limited views of who we think we are, and coming instead to know the true Self – and rendering the ego into service of it. Wilber (1998) writes: 'For authentic transformation is not a matter of belief but of the death of the believer; not a matter of finding solace but of finding infinity on the other side of death. The self is not made content, the self is made toast.'

A lifestyle 'guru' has become an essential prerequisite to happiness for many people (even, to much controversy, including the wife of the UK's prime minister in 2003). Having someone in your life to help you dress right, look right, speak right and act right is now as necessary as that not so subtly hidden designer label or the particular choice of holiday destination that is 'in' this year (Bennett, 2003). If evidence were needed of how we have degraded the guru concept, this is it.

True happiness is not brought about by shoring up the unending desire of our egos for power, prestige or personal wealth. The lifestyle guru, an oxymoron if ever there was one, is in the business (and a very expensive business it can be) of feeding the eternally hungry ghosts of our ego needs. The 'right lifestyle' in this context is light years away from, say, the 'right living' as preached by all the great spiritual teachers, including the founders of all the great faiths. There are common threads to be seen in both these perspectives. The lifestyle guru is shoring up the illusion of the self, pandering to it, fawning upon it, reinforcing it and at the same time nourishing its insatiable demands for satisfaction. The ego's desires are endless: give it one perfect dress it soon cries out for another; cut its hair 'just so' and it soon wants a change to be ahead of the pack; let it wallow in the perfect aromatherapy massage and it soon cries out for the next hit to make it feel better (and the same trick can apply if we get into drugs in the spiritual search; see Chapter 9). It can never get enough and the lucrative lifestyle market is tapping into this.

A real guru on the other hand does nothing to shore up the ego, but is in the business of aiding its demolition. The real guru does not feed the ego yet more to maintain its delusion of power and permanence, but starves it of all such nourishment until it collapses before an awareness of a deeper reality. They can do this safely with you because they have done it themselves. Such is the difference between the spiritual master and the lifestyle master. The one guides the stripping away of the ego's power so that we can come home to our true Self, the other keeps building it up with ever more alternatives in a (vain) attempt to keep it happy.

Such happiness is forever beyond our grasp. Pandering to this type of spiritual materialism leaves us always wanting more, a relentless hunt for contentment that is forever beyond our reach. Our TV channels are now flooded with programmes that testify to its unending demands, slot after slot dedicated to designing the perfect living room or choosing the perfect sweater or creating the perfect body. And all such desires must some day turn to dust. No matter what we reach for, we are certain to die, and no matter how much vanity we pile upon vanity, nothing can take that away.

All the great spiritual teachers, without exception, have pointed to the futility of this path and encouraged us to find happiness at a deeper, eternal level, which can only come from surrendering the ego demands and 'awakening to the inner reality of our being, to a spirit, self, soul which is other than our mind'. Such a path of surrender helps us 'to know, to feel, to be that, to enter into contact with the greater reality beyond and pervading the universe which inhabits also our own being' (Sri Aurobindo, 1970). Happiness does not come from feeding the ego, but from reducing its power to ashes!

Many healthcare staff like myself deal on a day-to-day basis with the exhausting search for happiness. Piling through our wards and clinics and outpatient departments are the endless queues of human misery often, in part at least, the product of the failed search. The exhausted, the depressed, the overweight, the underweight, the breathless, the ischaemic and so on are witness to the damage the search has wrought upon their bodies and minds. Some of us *might* end up as gurus, but meanwhile we have much to contribute as potential, positive lifestyle coaches ourselves, helping people to take better care of themselves. But we often fail our patients, not least because we may also have failed ourselves – not facing up to the fundamental ennui and despair that drives us for more when we may in fact need less. The true guru has worked on and with their ego, making it their servant not their master. When we come into their orbit, they call us to do likewise so that true happiness can be ours too. There's no avoiding this – the hard work has to be done. The spiritual search is no place for sissies!

No bypasses

In the plethora of New Age literature, workshops, experiential sessions, con-ferences and training programmes, there is an abundance of knowledge and ideas, and people only too willing to sell them to you. At their best, such peo-ple and events are authentic, rigorous, analytical and supportive of the seeker on their health and/or spiritual quest. At worst they are exploitative, manipu-lative and even downright dangerous. Both of these qualities can be found in the 'old age' belief systems too – the New Age phenomenon does not have a monopoly on either the best or worst approaches. The best 'walk their talk' of love, compassion, enlightenment; the worst may make the right noises, but do not live their lives accordingly – they have the talk but do not walk it in their everyday lives. The conference teacher sketched at the beginning of this chap-ter seems to fall into this last category.

There can be an unhealthy trap for the spiritual seeker and indeed for those who seek to guide them. The seeker can raise the shadow side in their teacher who, if they have not done the work on themselves, can be seduced by the desire for power and puffed-up self-importance over others. Just as the seeker may feed the ego of the mentor, so the teacher may consciously or uncon-sciously conspire to keep the student a good number of steps behind. The teacher continues to enjoy the power of their authority; the seeker or student gets somebody else take charge of things for them. The dance between seeker and teacher can itself be a spiritual practice, for example as the seeker learns to take responsibility for their own growing awareness and let go of their depend-ency on their 'master'.

> *Sometimes we can fall into thinking 'if I could only know enough, read the right books, do the right courses' then that would lead ipso facto into change in ourselves. Confronting our own demons and darkness – our anger, fear, desire, hatred and so on – these are the grist for the mill of the spiritual seeker. All the great spiritual paths agree that there is no spiritual search that does not include the call to confront the shadow, in all its forms, in ourselves.*
>   Wilber, 1991

The path requires us to bring into the light, as Wilber (1991) has indicated above, all our shadow side, to heal, resolve and integrate it.

> *In this war between opposites, there is only one battleground – the human heart. And somehow, in a compassionate embrace of the dark side of reality, we become bearers of the light. We open to the other – the strange, the weak, the sinful, the despised – and simply through including it, we transmute it. In so doing, we move ourselves toward wholeness.*
>
> Wilber, 1991

The mystics and spiritual seekers, ancient and modern, all agree that there are no short cuts, no bypasses (see St John of the Cross, 1973; Wolters (translator of *The Cloud of Unknowing*), 1978; Attar, 1984; Bankei, cited in Brandon, 1986; Harvey, 1991; St Theresa of Avila, 1995; Vaughan, 1995; Teasdale, 2001; Caplan, 2002). The road to enlightenment, to the Absolute, to closeness to the divine is the road through our own emotional swamp. There is no avoiding it. The work has to be done, for to do otherwise is to produce the false teacher, the false guru who talks right but does not live right, and unless they address the shadow they have sought to bypass, they may bring harm not only to themselves but to others. The person who sets themselves up as guru or teacher, perhaps aided by others who are themselves not fully awake and who conspire to elevate that person beyond their true depth, will from time to time leak the truth. Like my example, who lashed out at his wife and failed to pass the test.

SPOTTING THE FAKE AND STAYING HEALTHY

In previous chapters I have often emphasised the need for proper guidance on the spiritual quest, and Caplan (2002) and others affirm that, despite the risks, a guru is essential at some point for our safe, authentic spiritual awakening. When learning meditation, for example, we need to have the support in place of a wise person who has been there before us to engage with it safely. In Chapter 24 I will expand on wider support processes we can have in place to ensure the healthy exploration of our spirituality. How can we be sure that we are working with someone who is safe, when we are surrounded by so many tempting offers and people who seemingly 'know'?

One thing I have observed down the years is that teachers who are constantly telling you how fearful a place the world is, how much danger you are in, and often along with it implicitly or explicitly saying that you need to stick with them and follow them to be safe – these are the ones to avoid. All the great spiritual teachers down the years, whether they are theistic or atheistic, have one thing in common, the Absolute, the Ultimate Reality, the Transcendent, the Highest Self, God, is entirely loving in its manifestation.

In 2001 there was a terrible outbreak of foot and mouth disease in the UK. Huge numbers of animals were slaughtered and there was suffering and disruption in the community at many levels – especially among the rural community where I live. Apart from the three farms that border my home, you could travel for 50 miles around and not see a sheep anywhere. They were all consigned to fire or pit. I followed the story of the foot and mouth outbreak with particular interest for it directly affected the lives of myself and the people I live among. I recall being taken aback by a Radio 4 speech from a Church of Scotland minister who proclaimed the disease was a judgement of God for our bad farming practices. I felt dismay at such views; I would even describe them as a kind of blasphemy. Whether you believe in God or not, it seems a bit unfair to blame him/her/it for what is manifestly the product of human failings or even to presume that you know the mind of God at all. And even if it were a divine curse, what sort of loving God is it who zaps innocent animals for our misdemeanours?

What intrigues me here is the tendency of some individuals and religions to lapse into dogma whenever something fearful or uncertain is encountered. Fear makes some of us need fixed boundaries, ideologies or authority figures. In a fearfully uncertain world, some respond by surrendering themselves to others and some by demanding that everyone else conform to their world view (see Chapter 11).

Reverend Stephen Parsons (2000) has produced a fascinating thesis, which makes some uncomfortable reading for the Christian Church and which seems applicable to other faith groups as well. Religion and the spiritual search in the hands of certain people can damage your health. Nurses, doctors and other healthcare workers sometimes have to pick up the pieces of the victims, or may become one themselves. The nasty chemistry of co-dependence – when fearful people needing authority encounter fearful people seeking power – can produce all manner of abuse, as Parsons shows. Storr (1996) also did a demolition job on certain so-called gurus who abused their egomaniacal power over others, such as David Koresh, Jim Jones and Bagwan Shree Rajneesh to name but a few. Dogmatic thinking can be a harmless human frailty, but downright deadly amongst the vulnerable.

Storr, Parsons and others (e.g. Le Shan, 1974; Deikman, 1990; Vaughan, 1995) illustrate how easy it is for anyone to fall under the spell of the half-baked or self-appointed guru. When they have not done the work on themselves, the overweening power of their ego merely inflates itself, as Storr demonstrates, to ever more destructive heights – such as Jones' causing the massacre of hundreds of his followers in their South American enclave.

Our own vulnerability can draw us to such people – seeking those who can make life simple for us, give us certainty in an uncertain world. Yet, as Caplan (2002) has summarised, all the great spiritual teachings emphasise the value of the guru figure who, paradoxically, offers us the spiritual practice of surrendering to their authority for guidance. That surrender can be dangerous for those whose powers of discernment are limited or who are faced with an unscrupulous 'guru'. We can all be less discerning than usual, for example when bereaved or after certain spiritual practices such as long periods of fasting or meditation. However, a few checkpoints can give some protection, such as 'the Deikman test' – 'How does he treat his wife?' No matter how entrancing the guru or how many degrees in theology he holds, he betrays how much his fearful ego is still wrapped up in this stuff by the way he treats those near and dear to him. Put as much distance as you can between yourself and anyone who:

- does not walk their talk – preaching brotherly love, then damning to hell individuals and groups who differ from them
- asks you to abandon all critical thought and follow them blindly
- says that their knowledge is secret and can only be given to an elect few who have been initiated to their standards – can you imagine Jesus, Mohammed or the Buddha saying that their wisdom was secret?
- demands all your money, possessions, body etc.
- instructs you to get rid of all your relationships and activities not connected to the 'faith'
- runs an organisation that is really a big business
- tells you your lack of enlightenment is all your fault – you're not giving enough money, obedience, sex etc.
- is surrounded by bodyguards to keep followers remote
- has an organisation with pressure groups to make you conform rather than encouraging faith and trust
- commands that you remain in their sphere of influence, and not take what you need from them and move on.

If we follow a few pointers like these we may avoid the pitfalls of the ego-driven guru, especially in a world where so many seductive ones and their cults are so readily available (Barrett, 1996). When you next meet that great spiritual teacher or guru, just watch how they treat their partners, family or co-workers – watch very carefully.

CHAPTER 11

POURING OIL ON THE FIRE OF THE SOUL

Spill the oil lamp!
Set this dry, boring place on fire!
If you have ever
Made wanton love with God,
Then you have ignited that brilliant Light inside
That every person needs.
So —
Spill the oil!

Hafiz (translated by Ladinsky, 1996)

SUNDAY SCHOOL WITH GOD

I did not attend Sunday school for very long. I bunked off at the earliest opportunity in silent protest – a week of ordinary school followed by a Sunday session seemed too much like hard work. And the preacher in the Methodist Church was a bit of a hellfire and damnation type. I got to be scared spitless of God. And one Sunday it sank in; if He was everywhere and knew everything I did, then He was quite out of order. I grew up in a family where privacy was paramount and this applied particularly to the bathroom. So I remember well the long walk in the rain at the weekends to the toilet on my uncle's farm. It was an outdoor privy, not much more than a hole in the ground with a bench above it. And at seven years old I sat there with my grey flannel shorts around my feet hiding the holes in my socks and the scuffs on my tan sandals. I remember the sense of terror that this God who knew it all must be here too. But then I got to thinking that if God is in the loo with me, then He was just some kind of nosy parker who shouldn't be there. And Hey! Why should I pay attention anyway to some fat bearded bloke who lived in the sky and whose idea of fun was zapping people with lightning bolts every time they stepped out of line. And, anyway, my uncle, who said he didn't believe in God and that I shouldn't have anything to do with the churchmen and their lies, seemed to be a really happy man. As far as I could see the roof seemed unblasted by lightning and the toughest thing he ever seemed to experience was a bad chest in winter. And he was the kindest man I knew, who took me for long walks in the fields and taught me the ways of the animals, and how to pluck a chicken without suffocating with feathers, and how to help a sow in trouble give birth. He was at one with life, loved it, and some of that rubbed off on me. For quite a while, he became God to me.

HEALING OUR RELATIONSHIP WITH GOD – GETTING PAST THE FUNDAMENTALIST

One evening I was sat in quiet meditation with a friend, a paediatrician called Deb Lee, who is a committed Christian. Afterwards we spoke a little of our experiences of God and somehow got into a conversation around that fearful fundamentalist God who keeps popping up all over the place. (This ego-projected, rather nasty being recently and most visibly reared his ugly head as the Anglican Church tied itself in knots over a debate about the ordination of a gay bishop.) We both said, almost simultaneously, that this was not our experience of God. That hostile, damning, excluding imagery just did not fit with our experience of something that was profoundly loving, infinite and inclusive. Indeed we both felt a little dismayed by the way many faiths, not just Christianity, have hooked into this view. And how terribly wounding it can be.

As I write, I've just spent a few days with someone who, for a large part of her life, had been caught up in a fundamentalist religious sect. She has been terribly wounded by the experience and is now learning to cope with life, not least to make decisions for herself. The group and its leader give religion a bad name, and across the world we see the harmful and deeply unhealthy effects of people who believe their way is the right way and that everybody else should follow suit.

Religious fundamentalists are a curious group of people and I've worked with a few from time to time who are healthcare staff. They are curious because their fundamentalism is based on another 'F' word – fear. The fundamentalist finds the world a frightening place to be, full of contradiction, paradox and grey areas. They can't handle this, preferring the 'safe' territory of black and white, absolutes of right and wrong. If this were just their own stuff it might not be so bad, but the fundamentalist tends to extend this unhealthy control-freakery to others – friends and family, for example, damaging a lot of people's mental and spiritual health in the process (although they would see it as 'saving' them).

The second curiosity about fundamentalists is that, deep within, they don't *really* believe. Their certainty and absolutism is just a cover for an unconscious absence of faith. The fundamentalist would argue (sometimes violently) that this is not so, but of course it cannot be acknowledged simply because it is in the unconscious and not on the surface where it can be exposed to reason. Thus the fundamentalist will quote chapter and verse of scripture or stop their ears to open debate or different perspectives because even a scratching away at their surface veneer of righteousness can expose the denials, inconsistencies and, yes, essential lack of faith that lies beneath. Denial and defensiveness are crackingly good mechanisms for keeping uncomfortable reality, truth, at bay.

The biblical story of Jesus walking on the water (Matthew 14: 2–33) has a lesson for us here. The sea is stormy and Jesus walks out across the water to the disciples, terrified in the boat. He commands Peter to come to him. Peter does indeed set off walking on the water, until he gets scared and starts to sink. Jesus then grabs his hand and rescues him. Now, this story can be taken as a straight-forward testament to Jesus' supernatural state, putting him above and apart from the rest of us (not a view I personally share). But it can also be seen as a rich metaphor for the nature of faith. The security of the boat (religion, structure, certainty) has to be left behind at some point if we are truly to demonstrate faith in our beliefs, let go of our fear and take the risk of the waters of uncertainty. Religions, indeed belief systems in all their forms, are structures, which can (should) hold us safely, womb-like, until we are ready to move out of them into the wild waters of existence. Unfortunately we can sometimes be too scared (or not allowed) to let them go, limiting our capacity to fully experience life and relate to others, to really know ourselves and that which is beyond the self.

Fundamentalism takes many guises, not just religious or political, and it is always stifling of creativity and damaging to other human beings when it is acted out. There are even fundamentalist nurses, not in the religious sense, but in their beliefs about nursing. I met one prominent nurse theorist some years ago at a conference, who was quite clear that her nursing theory had all the answers. Nurses could dump the rest and find all they needed in hers. I listened patiently and took the first opportunity to head for the bar.

There's probably one you work with right now, the one who says, 'This is the way and it's the only way' or 'I've been doing it this way for 20 years and I'm not going to change.' Of course, this excludes yourself, dear reader, doesn't it? Things we believe in and do *may* be right, but the fundamentalist hangs on for fear of change; the true believer is open to question, to reason and to debate, and is willing to change when consistency is drowned by the greater power of truth.

Another person I would like to describe as an example of this process is Mark (not his real name), who had been coming to see me for a few months.

He had gradually shifted out of a very depressed and anxious state, dealt with all kinds of old childhood wounds and begun to revisit his latent connection to God. Like many people, he had been alienated from the greater realm of being, the Source, God, the Absolute, his deepest Self, call it what you will, because of the unholy (pun intended) alliance of a materialistic culture and the rigid dogma in at least some parts of the established faiths (in his case, Anglican Christianity).

Mark used the 'G' word, so for simplicity I will use it, too, from this point.

My job with him as his spiritual counsellor was to be with him while he sensitively and safely explored and re-visited his connection to God. He wanted to heal those wounds he had received in relation to God and religion. It was not my job to talk him into or out of God, but to help him find the wholeness he sought, from which he could confidently make the best decisions for himself. Very often people like Mark have become disconnected from God simply because of the bad experiences they have had with those in religious authority. Thus healing the relationship to God is often bound up with healing the old wounds inflicted by religion or other authority figures such as our parents. Miranda Holden (2002a) writes:

> Consciously or unconsciously, if your deepest perception of God is fearful, judgmental, conditioning or punishing, you will tend to be judgmental, conditional, punishing and fearful with yourself ... Your primal relationship to your God determines how you think of yourself. Unconsciously, you then project this dynamic onto everyone and everything. Holding onto a fearful image of God is not a good recipe for a happy and peaceful life.

I remember the day, during a period of prayer and meditation, that Mark saw at last, for himself, the falsity of that image of God, and I felt deeply honoured to be present with him when he finally connected with the love of God and not the fear. It has changed his life. The healing of his old wounds and his relationship to God were intimately bound up with each other.

THE SPIRITUAL COUNSELLOR HAS WALKED THE PATH ALREADY

There is much talk currently in the UK and elsewhere, now at government level even (see NHS Scotland, 2002; NHS England, 2003), encouraging a review of spiritual support services. It is interesting that such thinking is going on at government level – the disquiet that spiritual support for staff and patients in healthcare organisations (see Chapter 2) is not all that it could be seems to be edging policy-makers of health services into a lot of rethinking. One service, spiritual counselling, is often mentioned, yet there seems to be a real lack of clarity about what this role entails. Many books about conventional psychotherapy and counselling tend to embrace spirituality as a 'thing out there', a legitimate and rather late acknowledgement (despite the ground-breaking work of Jung and others) in the wider field of counselling, that spirituality, be it god-centred or not, is significant to clients (Young-Eisendrath & Miller, 2000; Griffith, 2002).

The objectification of spirituality goes some way towards helping our understanding of it, but I have been struck by how many manuals of guidance for therapists and counsellors concentrate on the spirituality of the client but largely ignore the spirituality of the counsellor. In the best traditions of 'physician heal thyself' it may be a very limiting form of counselling if the counsellor has not come to terms with their own wounds or understanding around the nature of God, the Absolute, the deepest Self, however they perceive it. Furthermore, a dualistic world is perpetuated – me counsellor, you client. Yet all forms of healing are a mutual process, as discussed in Chapter 19. It is this mutuality, this engagement with someone where barriers fall away that projects us into the safe sacred space from which healing emerges. This is holism, and holism and healing it may be recalled have the same linguistic and ontological roots.

Training opportunities for spiritual care and counselling are rare and variable in quality, and unlike the example of the Interfaith Seminary course in the UK, which is tough and rigorous (Porter, 2002), tend to focus on the spirituality of the client and how to 'talk about it'. Less attention is paid to what the spiritual outlook, needs and special skills of the carer or counsellor are. With the current encouragement in the UK for more health professionals to embrace spiritual support, my heart sinks at the thought that somebody somewhere will be setting up two-day workshops for nurses and other carers on how to give spiritual care.

Spirituality is not just a theory; it is a practice. Some of the most highly educated and experienced theologians I know are also the most cold and dogmatic people you could meet. Having done the training, be it a module on spirituality or subjecting oneself to being an ordinand in an established faith, is no guarantee of skills or knowledge in spirituality or, for that matter, personal holiness. In fact some of the most holy people I have known in my life have never been near a seminary or a faculty educational programme. I suspect our capacity to give spiritual support is directly proportional to our own level of spiritual awakening, and the latter is not achieved without tough personal work. It's not just about knowing the theory of different faiths and their customs, or embracing a few counselling skills, worthy as these might be in themselves. It is about an ever-deeper knowing of the self, and that which is beyond the self, that enables us to truly be with others in deep compassion and to put aside our own ego drives and agendas. All spiritual work is a kind of healing, and healing means going into the dark places of ourselves to heal our own wounds before we launch ourselves into the worlds of needy others. That way our spirituality becomes a truly embracing and loving practice, not a mask of good words or behaviour covering the shadows of our prejudices, phobias and bigotry.

Are there special qualities needed by those who engage in spiritual counselling? It could be argued that all that's needed is simply a heightened development of counselling skills and knowledge that's inherent in all healing relationships anyway. Furthermore, if we accept that all dis-ease, indeed disease, is primarily a product of disconnection from Source (*A Course in Miracles*, Anon., 1975) then the job of the counsellor is to be with people in such a way that they can reconnect to that Source. I am sceptical that this is possible unless the counsellor has him- or herself developed, and trusts in, a similar deep connection. Whatever that Source may be (and for me it is quite distinctly theocentric; although, as I have illustrated above, the healing had to be about resolving those old childhood distortions), it is this that is the ground of interplay between those who come for help and those who help.

One prerequisite for the spiritual counsellor seems to be that they are not hung up on the title. It's a useful phrase to help people find their way to the right source of help, although of course it may put some people off. Not everyone sees their problem as 'spiritual', and in view of the comments above about the wounds around God, it could indeed be an alienating title. I believe it was Jung who said that a problem before the age of 35 is a psychological one; after 35 it's spiritual. I'm not sure I would entirely agree with him about the dividing age but perhaps you see my point. It's often been my experience that the problem the client presents with is not really the problem. It is in the dance of their relationship with you that they may discover what has really drawn them to you.

Second, the spiritual counsellor has integrity. This includes their capacity to have integrated their own spiritual work and healing into their consciousness. They walk their talk and have become or are becoming the centred, Home-bound being in whose presence the other feels not overawed but safe and ready. They have walked the path that the spiritually needy person seeks, and having walked it before them, they have the knowledge, nay wisdom, that provides the safety net for the other to explore their spiritual landscape (Caplan, 2002; see also the previous chapter on the perils of false gurus, guides and teachers). The spiritual counsellor has not become attached to their title but has integrated the awareness that it is their function that matters. And it is their function to which they are dedicated, using all their spiritual practices to keep themselves in that heart-centred place of service to others. Integrity means 'standing for something', says Calhoun (1995). And this standing is more than the integration of parts of the self into a whole. It is 'fidelity to those projects and principles which are constitutive of one's core identity' – being in the world where their 'core', in Calhoun's words, is placed at the service of others.

Third, the spiritual counsellor does not get in the way. There is no struggle here to 'fix' the client by identifying their 'problems' and attempting to repair them (Guenther, 2002). The counsellor leaps across that limiting boundary line of healing. Resting in the trust of their own wholeness, their experience of the loving divine however it is manifested for them, they have no need to take anybody anywhere. Rather they hold the space, through prayer, meditation, visualisation or healing touch – whatever approaches are tested and intuitively arise for them – that holds the client while they make the opening to the Source, the deepest Self, for themselves. By keeping ourselves out of the way, the person can make that connection to God, the Absolute, however it is experienced for them. That connection can be made because no one stands, least of all the helper, between them and the Source they seek and which, some would argue, seeks them. The helper/counsellor stays out of the way because at a deep level they are not in control of the process – they may participate in it as a sort of spiritual midwife, but the process is essentially a natural one and the person is birthing that which they already contain. Note how we use words like 'reveal', 'discover', 'reawaken' in soul work. These words (like dis-cover for example) suggest that what is emerging is not new, rather it is inherently present, waiting to be released. In our deepest selves we already 'know', all we have to do is recall (re-call) it.

For many conventional therapists, rooted in the certainty that, armed with their therapeutic tools, they are very much in charge, the idea that they really are not may be scary. 'It is not so much about knowing all the right answers as knowing all the right questions', as one friend said to me. The questions, sensitively placed at the right location, can be a kind of cattle prod to the consciousness, provoking it to wake up and really *see*, to open up and be willing to *receive* – what? Call it what you will – God, awareness, love, light, the greater realm of being, truth. The counsellor simply points the way, holds the space and leaves the rest to the unknown and only partially knowable, to God, or to the 'holy presence' as Guenther (2000) describes it. The counsellor does nothing but sit patiently waiting and alert, offering a word or a gesture that comforts or challenges and holding the client while they birth their own connection. Doing nothing except the hard work of keeping out of the way can paradoxically be an effortless effort. There is no sacrifice, no labour, because the counsellor does not have to be in charge. Nothing is done and nothing is left undone.

Spiritual counselling in this context is a mutual process; the other does not move alone and we cannot stay without the ground of our own experience of the divine. Where I am is intimately bound up with where you are and where we both might be. Spiritual counselling is prayer in action. It is the performance of miracles because we do not control the performance and because the outcome can transcend the normal boundaries of what can be expected or always understood.

A FINAL REMINISCENCE

Sorting out God for ourselves is a primary requisite of the helper of those (all?) with spiritual helping needs. Oddly enough it has personally taken me quite a while to get used to the 'G' word. I feel OK with it now, but it has been a long time getting there. Getting past all the labels and what they conjure up has been a hard task – tough spiritual work indeed. I remember an incident maybe ten years ago now, about the time I was 'waking up'. For some reason I'd got myself into an intellectual tailspin about the nature of God. At that time I was still struggling with the very possibility of his/her/its existence. (It took me a long time to learn that the way in was not via my head but the heart, but thereby hangs another tale.) I left the house and went to sit in my favourite meditation spot. It was late evening and the end of a warm spring day. I decided in my arrogant determination that I was going to do a Buddha – I had a question to be answered and I was going to sit out there and not move until I got it. I remember saying aloud (I live in the country – it was safe to talk to myself; had I been in the town they would have carted me off to the nearest psychiatric clinic, I'm sure!), 'OK, if you exist at all, I want some answers. Who are you? Are you a he or a she or an it? Let's start with that one. I'm not moving until I get an answer even if they find me dead here in a week's time. I'm going nowhere until I know.' What happened next is the stuff of mysticism or madness: I leave you, dear reader, to choose. All I can say is that I heard a voice 'in my head' quite clearly saying, 'I am all and neither. Call me whatever you want, see me in whatever way you want, it doesn't matter to me. Call me anything. Call me a duck if you want to.' At that precise moment, with a clatter of wings a pair of ducks rose up in the air from the overgrown ditch behind me and quacked their way over my head and down into the field before me. I broke into laughter and went indoors to make myself a cup of cocoa. Ever since then I've kept a little wooden duck in my meditation room at home, though I rarely tell anyone why! I remember Stan Grof's precautionary advice on spiritual awakening – to be very careful about what you say and to whom. What to you is wise and inspiring, may be the stuff of psychosis to others.

God is such a little word for something so full of paradox, so full of teasing concepts, unnameable, faceless yet with every name and every face. Immanent and transcendent, remote and intimate, containing everything, being no-thing. Far greater sages and scholars have tried to define the indefinable. For myself and my friend Deb – it's just lovingly, inexhaustibly *there*. But that's my view; others might differ. Yet it is the very ground of the relationship on which we stand when the needy come for help. And we stand or sit, ready to 'pour on the oil', not in a proselytising or dogmatic or instructing way, just in a loving, present way that allows the person to find their own way Home. And Home can be many things to many people – a deep loving acceptance of themselves and others, a true forgiveness of the past, a growing connection with God in whatever form, a capacity to be increasingly compassionate in the world for themselves and others.

However it manifests itself, the end product of successful spiritual counselling, if there is one, is a more well-rounded human being, more connected, more at one and at home in themselves and their God, their soul and their deepest selves. Their capacity to be in the world is more expansive yet more grounded, more available yet more integrated, and more 'alive' yet more focused. Pouring on the oil has ignited their own true self – never to be extinguished.

CHAPTER 12

GIVE ME DARTH VADER ANY DAY – THE BLESSING OF EGO WORK

One does not become enlightened by imagining figures of light, but by making the darkness conscious.

Jung, 1961

NEW AGE FLUFFINESS

I get lots of love and light. They arrive at the end of email missives, tagged on to postcards from abroad, slipped into Christmas greetings. I appreciate what friends and loved ones are trying to say. They wish me wellness and happiness, a life full of joy, contentment and bliss. I wouldn't want to gainsay that or to suggest that their good wishes and prayers are unwelcome or unappreciated. As prayer and non-local healing seem to work, as discussed in Chapter 5, then I'll take all I can get, thank you.

But occasionally, just occasionally, and in the knowledge that our consciousness, our deepening spiritual awareness, is formed not in love and light but in an often painful exploration of our shadow side, I hope that they would wish me darkness. It is in my shadow that I learn, confronting all those parts of the self – anger, fear, lust, hurt and so on – that many people would perhaps rather keep quietly hidden away. It is here that I am burnished, where the alchemical process of the soul does its work. Darkness and shadow are the places in my soul where hammer and anvil forge my way of being in the world. Without it there is no contrast, no medium for creation, no opportunity.

In most Western cultures, to willingly enter those shadow places of ourselves is often seen as a kind of spiritual suicide. Surely, our job is to hold ourselves always in light, avoid darkness and always seek a world full of niceness and kindness. Unfortunately, that doesn't seem to work. Efforts to avoid our shadow side only seem to strengthen it. We fall into denial, permitting some of the worst atrocities to be committed in the name of love and light. When the shadow side of our natures and organisations is not worked on, when we attempt to bypass it by rigid adherence to apparent rules and lifestyles based on light and love, we risk projecting it outwards. In doing so we may end up plunging others and ourselves into all manner of abuse and danger, as Stephen Parsons' (2000) work indicates.

In our search for the sacred, not least in ourselves, there is a common tendency to want blissful experiences, full of light and love, and to turn away from the mundane, the nasty or what we see as darkness or evil. This applies to what we see as the darkness in ourselves, as well as in the rest of the world. It is relatively easy to look at the wider world with all its shadows and pain, much more difficult to turn the roving eye inward and see what dark shadows may lurk within ourselves. However, if we are to enter into right relationship with others and the wider world, we must also embark upon that voyage of self-discovery to enter right relationship with ourselves and all the light and shadow that lies at the very heart of each and every one of us.

Throughout the ages, in many spiritual teachings, from the Upanishads to the Bible, from the Sufi and Christian mystics of the Middle Ages to Buddhist past and present teachers such as Bankei or Jack Kornfield, much the same message is conveyed – that light and dark exist in all things; that both are sources of soul work; that all is part of the One, the Creator, the Absolute, God, Ultimate Reality; and that the union of the two forces through acceptance and compassion is a universal goal. In becoming a unified whole, that same goal for each human being presents itself – to work with not only the light and love in ourselves, but also our shadow side.

The joy and pain of life, reflected in the human condition, is all part of the oneness of life. The light and the dark are present in each of us. That struggle with the darker part of ourselves is well illustrated in the hero's journey in many elements of popular culture, both ancient and modern, from Persephone's journey into the underworld and the epic Persian story of Gilgamesh, to Luke Skywalker's struggle with himself in the *Star Wars* series and the heroic fellowship of the nine in the *Lord of the Rings* saga. These stories contain essentially the same elements – the heroes' entry, willingly, into darkness in order to return with the light. It is worth remembering that what makes the legends so thrilling and enduring is not just the goodies who win, but the figures of shadow. Without the likes of Darth Vader or Sauron, they would be dreadfully dull stories. For Jesus it was the struggle against Satan, for the Buddha it was the challenge of composite evil, the Mara. In Egyptian mythology it is the war between Horus, the divine messenger between heaven and earth, and his brother Seth, wielder of dark forces of anger and revenge.

Such archetypes inform us of the nature of the endless human struggle between the light and dark in each of us. They also illustrate that the challenge is also to move beyond the duality of light and dark — towards wholeness, towards union. Each must accept the existence of the other as a necessary part of the creation. All the darker parts of the self are but grist for the mill; they are teachers, things to work with as we follow the road that leads to deeper understanding of the self. However, so often we seek to bury our darker side in the belief that, if we ignore it, it will go away or at least lose its influence over us. The opposite seems to be the case. To do spiritual work, to discover the sacred within ourselves, we cannot bypass the emotional work. All of the great spiritual teachers down through the ages sought not to bury their darker sides, but to work with them, suffer with them and bring them into the light.

However, I have attended so many gatherings, meetings and New Age and 'old age' events where everyone appears happy and shiny and smiley, but where this is just a front, a mask placed over the face that dare not show itself. David Steindl-Rast (1991) writes of the 'New Age' searchers for whom 'The shadow has been conspicuous by its absence. Seekers often are led to believe that with the right teacher or the right practice, they can transcend to higher levels of awareness without dealing with the more petty vices or ugly emotional attachments.' Marc Barash (1993) is equally scathing: 'Spirituality, as repackaged for the New Age, is a confection of love and light, purified of pilgrimage and penance, of defeat and descent, of harrowing and humility.' Many would argue that it is not just the New Age that tends to succumb to this denial of the shadow. A tuning in to many current radio and TV programmes can reveal a similar tendency to fall into saccharin sweetness and avoidance of the bitter aspects of religion and spirituality.

John Babbs (1991) writes:

> I went last night, as I have so many other nights, to one of those wondrous New Age gatherings. And I don't think I can take any more. I get sick. I must escape the torture of being blessed to death during evenings such as this. There is something frighteningly unreal about them that I can't quite put my finger on. All I know is that afterwards I want to scream profanities, drink whiskey out of a bottle, go to sleazy blues joints and chase wild, wild women. At this event a beautiful young man told of his travels throughout the globe visiting sacred ceremonial sites — four hundred all told. He has been around the world 14 times in his 34 years, living in many of these places for months, sometimes years on end.

Sometimes leaving our ordinary lives is necessary to experience the extraordinary. To then integrate this more fully into our way of being, transforming our everyday lives and relationships, would seem to be a healthy approach to retreat. Dropping out in order to avoid experiencing the pain of the world seems a dead end. Becoming a spiritual tourist in search of more 'highs' has just the same addictive, avoiding quality to it of the attachment to the entheogens described in Chapter 9.

ALCHEMY

The ancient art of alchemy is often reduced to a view of strange men in even stranger clothes, dabbling in magic in an effort to turn lead into gold in pursuit of great riches. We need to look at the story as metaphor, of finding ways to turn the shadowy leaden parts of ourselves into the golden possibilities of illumination and awareness. The stories of alchemists are echoed in the Arthurian legends in pursuit of the Holy Grail. Working with all the darkness of the world, the Knights of the Round Table seek the chalice believed to have been used by the Christ himself. Again we can see a metaphor at work here, replicated in myths and stories around the world throughout the ages – the heroic journey into darkness to discover a great treasure or fire. Perhaps the reward should be seen not so much as earthly riches or power, but as self-discovery and enlightenment.

In his modern fable *The Alchemist*, Paolo Coelho's (1993) heroic boy hears the whispering of his heart which says, 'Be aware of that place where you are brought to tears. That's where I am, and that's where your treasure is.' In other words the alchemy of the spiritual quest is turning darkness into light, coming into loving acceptance of ourselves. The greatest heroic journey that each of us can undertake is that where we enter our own shadow, reveal it, and thereby turn it to light – the discovery of our own holy grail. Exploring the sacred in ourselves means that we must look at all the parts of ourselves; alchemy requires all the elements to turn lead into gold. Such an integration is integral to our own health, our own right relationship with ourselves and perhaps our God.

Such an integrative process affects not just ourselves, but everything around us. As we shift our view of the world and our place in it, there is a knock-on effect in our work, our relationships, our interests and so on. As we turn more into light, others around us cannot avoid being affected by it. Coelho also writes, 'When we strive to become better than we are, everything around us becomes better too.' Andrew Harvey (1991), documenting his spiritual awakening and especially his challenging contact with Mother Meera (an Indian woman, currently based in Germany, who offers spiritual guidance, believed by many to be an 'avatar', a divine, realised being working on earth), adds: 'No awakening can be personal or selfish. Every awakening spreads its power and light throughout the world.' If we take Watson's (1980) report on the 'hundredth monkey' to its logical conclusion, the implications of a mass of people awakening spiritually are enormous. In this study, the learning of one group of monkeys seems to have been transmitted to others without any social contact with the other groups. With no obvious physical communication between them, it seems that other groups of monkeys were able to learn from the first group once a critical mass of understanding had been achieved in that group. By some process we do not fully understand (and similar experiments have been conducted with other animals) it seems that a wider change can occur, once enough individuals shift their way of being in the world in some way.

Thus the notion of our own work, healing and coming home to ourselves, of transforming darkness into light, has an impact upon others. In *The Garden of the Prophet*, Kahlil Gibran (1933) says, 'So shall the snow of your heart melt when the spring is come, and thus shall your secret run in streams to seek the river of life in the valley. And the river shall enfold your secret and carry it to the great sea . . .' In the spring, which comes shedding new light on our cold dark places, we melt to join the sum total of the conscious river of humanity. Our change makes change in the whole.

A WORD OF CAUTION

Working on our shadow does not mean that we have to abandon ourselves to the pit of danger and despair if we are to pursue our understanding of our spirituality. The path should be approached with care and caution. *The Cloud of Unknowing* (translated by Wolters, 1978), believed to be a late seventeenth-century text on the spiritual journey by an unknown author, reminds us that we should 'Be careful in this matter, and do not overstrain yourself emotionally or beyond your strength. Work with eager enjoyment rather than with brute force. The more eager your work, the more humble and spiritual it becomes.' Making the more difficult path a source of learning seems to be the object lesson in confronting the shadow in ourselves. Thus we become alchemists of the soul, transforming lead into gold. In the shadow there is danger, but also hope.

James Jones (1996), a psychotherapist and professor of religion, points out:

> *Dangerous? Yes, but equally dangerous is a life without ecstasy, without the numinous, without depth, breadth, passion, meaning or purpose. Spirituality is process before content. Not memorising rules, facts or concepts, but freeing the mind and the heart to explore new worlds of insight.*

So, fear of the shadow side of ourselves, and of exploring it, may keep us from entering into right relationship with ourselves, others and perhaps our God. Right relationship in other arenas of our lives is underpinned by right relationship with the self. The strength of our fearful egos, shored up by the endless wounds we have received in life, can make it difficult for us to risk the long hard look at ourselves through the window of our soul into the shadow that lurks there. Yet, if we are to be of service to others, it is to ourselves that we must look first. The path of life has left none of us unscathed or unwounded, and this applies no less to those involved in caring for others. Very large numbers of professional and informal carers are themselves 'co-dependent' or bringing their own difficulties into the caring relationship, however unconsciously, as we have seen. Healing the wounded healer is part of the work of those who seek to care for and heal others. Zwieg & Adams (1991) remind us that the healing of the healer takes place in the integration of shadow and light within. Thus healed, we become infinitely more available to the healing of others.

The notion of each of us contributing to the diminution of the darkness by working on ourselves is repeated by Robert Bly (1991) who says:

> So the person who has eaten his shadow spreads calmness and shows more grief than anger. If the ancients were right that the darkness contains intelligence and nourishment and even information, then the person who has eaten some of his or her shadow is more energetic as well as more intelligent.

An exploration of our own darkness is an essential part of our spiritual awakening. It is critical to those who work in caring relationships with others if they are to let go of their own co-dependencies, needs for power and other potential sources of abuse of the sick and the vulnerable. A start on that journey is the recognition of the darkness in ourselves, not as something to be avoided but to be welcomed as a valued teacher, indeed friend – the grist for our mill where shadow can be transmuted, with caution and support, into light. Scary as it may be, we can offer it a welcome and acknowledge it for all it has to teach us.

SPIRITED LEADERSHIP

All this talk of integrating the shadow would be so much theory, were it not for the consequences when we do not, especially of we are in positions of power. And every healthcare worker has immense power over those who are diseased and dis-eased, as do those in management and leadership positions over their teams. The following vignette concerns someone I worked with a couple of years ago who held a very senior position managing a hospital.

He was a nice enough person, quite affable, a good sense of humour, passionate about health care and determined to go places. He wanted the top job, to be in charge of a hospital some day, so that all his vision for what an excellent service could be would be realised. And yet here he was, in retreat here at the Sacred Space Foundation, close to burnout and full of anger and resentment and vengeance. He railed against colleagues who didn't seem to work as hard as he did, who 'swung the lead' and deserved some harsh discipline, who ought to be cleared out if they got in his way. At the same time he had a gentle, compassionate side, really wanting to nurture colleagues into doing their best, enabling and empowering them – shadow and light in one man, as in all men (and women).

We talked a lot about what life would be like when he finally made it to the top. He was aware of that part of his nature that could be bruising towards others but was quite convinced that, once he got into a position of power, he wouldn't need to worry about it, or others. Freed of restraints, he would be able to be the kind of boss he would have liked to have had himself – supportive and encouraging. His best side, he believed, would be able to come to the fore and he would produce a wonderful 'magnet' organisation where staff would love to be. He was quite angry with me when I suggested that maybe it wouldn't be that simple. Just as there was every possibility that a new role with more power would bring out the best in him, so it was equally likely that it would give even greater free rein to the worst in him, too.

Much more attention is being paid these days to leadership development in the UK health services and, I know from my travels in many countries across Europe, North America and Australasia, that the same applies there. I hope these programmes will have learned from the approaches to leadership in the past. So often we have modelled healthcare leadership and management development on theories borrowed from social psychology and industry. These often do little to challenge underlying notions of power and control, and the subject of spirituality barely gets a look in. Yet, as we examined in Chapter 2, there is increasing evidence that organisations that attend to the spiritual needs (meaning, purpose, connection, involvement) of the staff are more likely to be successful.

I've been working with some senior clinical nurses recently, all of them pushing back the boundaries of practice. It is interesting to see the positive, 'can do' attitude that emerges from those who come from nurturing workplaces contrast with the oppressed, embattled view that comes from those who have to work with bosses who are heavily controlling. The latter type of boss essentially operates on a basis of fear – they rule others for fear of loss of control, of their own jobs, their prestige, their power, their lives. Once again we encounter the end product of people in power acting out their shadow side. They have got to the top, but have bypassed the emotional and spiritual work on themselves. Such an approach to leadership is a world away from that advocated by groups such as the servant-leader network (Spears, 1998), which is heavily influenced by Quaker spirituality. This recognises that leaders are not just involved in controlling others; they also concern themselves with nurturing and serving them to be the best people they can be, totally involved in the goals of the organisation. Spears and others postulate that such leaders cannot emerge unless they have embraced all dimensions of themselves, have learned to let go of models of leadership based entirely on power and control, and have come to rest with more equanimity in the world.

Such leader-managers are a joy to work with. They may have done the usual outward-bound course in their management development, but they have also committed themselves to inward-bound work as well. Their spiritual work provides them with an easier connection with themselves, their work and all that is, whether their cosmological view is god-centred or not. People who are comfortable with themselves and their place in the scheme of things have much less fear dogging their lives and they are much less likely therefore to dump their fears on others. Health care needs more spirited leaders.

SEDUCED BY THE SHADOW OF OUR OWN MYTHOLOGY

Seduction, telling ourselves that shadow is really light, is another neat trick of the ego, to boost our sense of worth and tell ourselves that we are OK, really, and that what we are doing, even if it is patently wrong, is really right. An example of this has stuck in my mind for a couple of years now.

I must have walked several yards out of the office before I stopped myself and heard myself saying, 'She said hospice! I'm sure she said *hospice*.' I doubled back on myself and went to my directory and, sure enough, there it was. The trustee I had just spoken to, and from whom I had heard a long tale of alleged damage and disruption to patients and staff, was representing a hospice.

It says something about my own conditioning that I would have had no problem accepting the tales of bullying and harassment of staff and substandard care to patients had the person I'd just spoken to worked in the mainstream NHS. The long list of hospital enquiries down the years has accustomed me to expect failures, often severe ones, from time to time. My work these days revolves a lot around conflict resolution and from time to time I have been asked to conduct enquiries into settings where things have gone badly wrong. But never before in a hospice.

There is, of course, no logical reason why a hospice should not experience problems like any other workplace, but I recognised instantly in myself that I had internalised certain assumptions about caring settings like hospices. Those assumptions were about to be challenged as the enquiry got under way, followed by the shattering consequences of the results (allegations of bullying and harassment proven; failures in clinical leadership and standards of care uncovered; many staff moved on or disciplined or dismissed). The hospice – yes, a hospice – had declined into what was in effect classic institutionalised behaviour. A significant number of staff across disciplines had come to see the hospice as existing to meet their needs, and the patients, the raison d'être of the hospice, were like a drama playing off set somewhere in another theatre. The staff, at least most of them, had not arrived at this point consciously. Oh no, in that sense, they were not 'bad' people. They had not deliberately (or at least with a couple of exceptions) set out to make trouble or neglect their responsibilities to their colleagues and patients – far from it, and I suspect that most of those who were dismissed or disciplined will go to their graves thinking that they were right and were unjustly accused. Only rarely did one or two staff have the insight and awareness to see what had gone wrong and confront it in themselves. Further, they then demonstrated considerable courage in some instances not only in facing their own demons, but also in sticking to the truth and right action even though it meant putting their careers and their colleagues' in jeopardy.

In this deeply dispiriting environment, right relationships at many levels had collapsed, and were it not for a few enlightened, indeed brave, managers and staff, that sick institution would be continuing its course to this day. Don't get me wrong; the place wasn't a complete disaster, as most patients got through the system with modestly good care, but in the case of a few where it went wrong it went badly wrong, and the undercurrent of risk (e.g. not following acceptable drug error policies) was an accident waiting to happen. The place is much recovered and continuing to do so, but dialogues I have had in recent years with a great many hospice staff lead me to believe that this particular site is not alone — it's just that a lot of them aren't prepared to face up to the issues yet. Time will tell.

The problem starts when we lose sight, for whatever reason, of the core purpose and meaning of our work. The distorted vision draws us away from reality into a world governed by our own over-inflated self-importance. We internalise false beliefs in ourselves ('We work with the dying, we are kind, we are caring'), reinforced when patients and public alike assure us of how wonderful we are, how marvellous we must be to do such a job because 'I could never do it.'

All of us can experience these sweet seductions at some stage and we can shrug them off for what they are: well-meaning but essentially vacuous comments. But they can become lethal if we take them on board to reinforce some co-dependent shadow quality in us — the need to be needed, to feel powerful, to feel wonderful. Multiple checks and balances need to be in place to maintain constant vigilance — such as appraisal, reflective practice, a constant questioning of values and beliefs (and, yes, this includes our spiritual practice), effective leadership, quality assurance programmes and so on. Otherwise, like these particular hospice staff, we fall into the seduction of the mythology about ourselves — nurses and doctors are wonderful, the patients' and public's 'We could never do that.'

Sometimes this collective denial, masked by the myth of our own goodness, allows the most terrible horrors to be perpetrated under our very noses, simply because we cannot believe that 'one of us' would do it. Indeed, I remember the enquiry into Bev Allitt, the nurse who killed many children in the early 1990s. One element there, which allowed the perpetrator to continue her destructive behaviour, was that members of the staff were even prepared to believe in curses and evil spirits rather than consider the awful truth that the shadow was quite human: one of their own was responsible (Davies, 1993).

No setting is immune to this grand seduction. Beware of the siren call that tells us 'We are ever so wonderful.' We are all in shadow to some degree, both individually and collectively. The bulwarks against the worst effects are a relentless vigilance and layer upon layer of individual and collective practices (including our spiritual practices) and policies, which keep the truth of ourselves and our work exposed to the cool light of day, and provide us with the opportunity to transmute shadow to light.

CHAPTER 13

THE CINEMA OF THE SOUL – PROJECTIONS OF SHADOW AND LIGHT

How could there be so much evil in the world?
Knowing humanity, I wonder why there is not more of it.

Hannah and Her Sisters, Woody Allen

WARRIORS OF LIGHT AND DARK

When I was a small boy, I managed to avoid large tracts of school life by being sick. In quick succession between the ages of 5 and 7 I contracted measles, mumps, whooping cough, scarlet fever and chicken pox. In fact, I remember being taken by my mum to visit a friend who had chicken pox. My mother, to my knowledge, had no sadistic tendencies; it was just what you did in those days. As soon as one kid popped up with one of the perennial infections, the mums would ensure rapid contact to make sure that all their children got whatever it was as well. It was, of course, a traditional way of dealing with infections and preventing more serious problems later in life – making sure the kids all got it soon and built up an immune response. People knew that risking a nasty illness was worth it for longer-term benefits.

I remember those sick days and nights well – especially the raging fevers and the nightmares. My nightmares were all ones of crushing claustrophobia, and in my terror and sweat I remember surrendering into the arms of my mum when she climbed into bed and held on to me until the fear passed. My body was learning about disease through willing exposure – and how to resist it by acquiring knowledge of that disease itself.

Nowadays in Western culture there is a tendency to avoid dirt and disease of any kind. Suffering is not what we are supposed to do. This avoidance reaches out into so many New Age, and not so New Age, spiritual offerings where the experience should be one of sweetness and light. A confection of bliss is offered and the shadow, in whatever form, is to be avoided at all costs, as we have explored in Chapter 12. The 'shadow' in all its forms, from the personal pain and suffering of life to the Jungian individual and collective unconscious to the notions of evil and demonic forces and on to the darkness that is the void – the place that is no place yet pregnant with the possibilities of creation. And perhaps something beyond that which is dark and yet not dark.

Rilke (translated by Bly, 1981) offers a perspective that the darkness is perhaps not entirely to be feared when he writes of it as the place of human origin, the place where a 'great energy' gathers and in which he has 'faith'. The darkness we so much fear is perhaps also our greatest teacher.

I have lost track of the number of emails I get that warn me about the darkness that is enveloping the world. Usually full of doom-laden scenarios, they offer apocalyptic visions (dressed up in new words but offering the same ideas recycled) of a selected few who will be saved if only they follow certain spiritual practices or beliefs. They usually go something like this – the Earth is a battleground between the forces of light and dark. This battle is about to come to a head on . . . (insert the date of your choice here). The light warriors will be saved, the rest have had it, and the earth will return to its original state of paradise. This archetypal vision often says much more about our fearful projections onto an uncertain world and a limited, reductionist view of the divine 'plan' than it does about the reality of planetary history. It denies the possibility that such views through the lens of paranoia may fall short of the endless possibility (and optimism) of the creation. The vision tends to incorporate a rather nasty, authoritarian and punishing God, a regimented approach to salvation – only if you do certain things will you be saved and a fairly puffed-up perspective of humanity on this planet as being the epicentre of all that is.

A glance through any newspaper could give the impression the world is indeed on a hiding to nothing. Filled with murder, mayhem and madness, from mass slaughter to environmental crisis – we can be forgiven for thinking that maybe we have lost the plot and the game is very much up. I'm not so sure that it's ever been any different. With modern technology we just get to know more about it, and because we get to know more about it, therein lies hope.

UNHEALTHY PROPHETS – FEAR AND LOATHING ON THE INTERNET

I had another example in my inbox a few months ago, but this time the message was subtly different. It's not so much that the idea that humanity is doomed represents a projection outward of all our fears; rather this time it is a projection outward onto some other authority figure that it's all going to be OK because somebody/God is about to sort it all out for us. They pop up in mailshots and New Age journals and whizz round the Internet – the elements vary, but the essential nature is the same. Some person/persons are telling us that now is the time of transformation of human consciousness, the dawn of a New Age, the coming of the great spiritual teachings/guardians that will solve all of our problems. Humanity is going to come into perfection at this time, now, next week, within the year, etc.

I suppose it's wise to keep an open mind to these things, but I see so many of them and your average bookstore's 'mind-body-spirit' shelf is sighing under the weight of New Age and not so New Age prophecies. But, as my teacher Ram Dass once told me, keeping an open mind doesn't mean you have to empty your head.

I'm inclined to treat the phenomenon not as prophetic visions but as ego-driven delusions. They tap into a lucrative market – one built on our desire in a scary world for hope, certainty, safety, specialness, power. Courses, books, journals, subscription websites and so on generate income from this triumph of human frailty over reason. Much of it is fluffy and harmless, but some can be downright dangerous, sucking people into cults and under the spell of dubious gurus. And all of it is usually expensive.

Gimme a break. First of all, can you imagine a real prophet (a Jesus, Buddha, Krishna, Mohammed, Guru Nanak) offering to enlighten us and relieve our suffering, but telling us we have to pay for it first? Can you imagine any of them saying that what they had to offer was for the elite few as opposed to the whole of humanity? Can you envision any of them suggesting that a single human being or group of human beings was going to take charge of the cosmic order and sort it out for us?

Spinning these prophetic webs is also fundamentally disempowering. We are being asked to sign up to somebody else's control and plan for the world, another's solution as an easy spiritual quick fix, instead of surrendering to the tougher work of exploring what is in our own hearts and arriving at our own solutions. The former approach means we can escape from the swampy low-lands, the messy and difficult terrain of our own soul exploration, and hand the problem over to a ready-mix prescription. This is especially seductive if what is being offered is a saccharin fairytale promise that warms the cockles of your heart and leaves out the whelks of everyday life.

There seem to be so many psychic beings around these days, putting the world to rights, that if they were really as good and god-sent as they are cracked up to be, we would already be living in nirvana. Well, we're not and I suspect we may never be, least not while attached to this reality. Its very nature may be its contradictions, its joys and its sorrows, its loves and its labours – it is as it should be to provide us with the test bed of our psyches, the grist for the mill for the evolution of our soul and consciousness.

A friend of mine sent me a rather nervous-sounding note in response to one of these prophetic emails. Should he really be following this sort of thing up? Might he be missing something? He was sceptical, he said, but was anxious that there might be something in it. I suggested that he rested with his scepticism; having a good spiritual 'bullshit-detector' is an invaluable asset in the current spiritual hypermarket. I have a feeling that if heaven on earth really does arrive (and actually from my point of view, it is in the here and now if we would but open to it), the prophets would be well pissed off! It seems important to suss out these unhealthy spiritual profferings for what they are – a response to our deep-seated neuroses. When they've been rumbled, they might see not only that heaven has been opened to all, but also that neither they nor their devotees have got front-row seats.

Of course, I could be completely wrong, in which case I've missed out on enlightenment, the second coming and the answer to the meaning of life for the third time this week. Damn. Never mind, there's always another shift.

DARKNESS MASKING AS LIGHT

Like motherhood and apple pie, some things are so self-evidently good and true that to challenge them consigns you to the realms of the insane or the criminal. But terrible things can sometimes be done in the name of goodness and truth.

I recall watching a Channel 4 programme on Afghanistan, where a religious leader of the Taliban enthused about the slaughter of men because they were homosexual, of women because they breached codes of conduct. Kidnappers in Iraq have beheaded their hostages as I write. Terrorists corrupt a profound Islamic concept – jihad – into holy war, when jihad is really more concerned with the inner struggle of the soul to reach truth, not bombing and gunblasting your way through those who disagree with or have offended you. Things done in the name of a limited and ignorant interpretation of Islam like this horrifies most Moslems as deeply as non-Moslems. Such distortions fuel the current demonising of Islam.

When we create absolutes of truth, we can separate from us those who deviate from 'our' truth. If our way is good, then theirs must be bad. Disconnecting from our fellows thus, we can ultimately do whatever we want to them. Not like us = less human than us.

This is all another neat ego trick we use to convince ourselves that we are OK. We can do all manner of things to people in the name of righteousness or justice by convincing ourselves that all the wrong in the world exists in others and not ourselves. I attended a meeting of thousands of nurses recently at the annual congress of the Royal College of Nursing, followed by meetings of some of our major political parties. On the basis of some of what I witnessed, these membership groups should be charging therapy fees to their members for the service they provide – allowing large numbers of people to feel better by having a go at the leadership or other people for being 'wrong'.

Making ourselves feel bigger by making others feel smaller is one of the oldest ego tricks in the book. From time to time, it can take more sinister turns when individuals, indeed whole cultures, project their shadow onto other individuals and groups. And 'other' is the key word – by separating ourselves from other humans we can dehumanise them, allowing us to perpetrate all manner of horrors. The twentieth-century conflicts in Rwanda and Bosnia, and the holocaust of the Nazi era, are classic examples of what happens when we project our shadow on to others.

It's happening now in conflicts all across the world. Nothing to do with us? It's only a question of degree. I have worked in a super cultural and educational institute in the delightful village of Irsee, not far from Munich. The exquisitely renovated building was a religious foundation with a hospital attached. Some 2000 people died here during the war from the willing actions of (Christian) nurses and doctors who, in the service of the 'greater good', thought it right to help rid Germany of 'life not worth living' ('lebensunwertes Leben') (Lifton, 1986; Goldhagen, 1997).

Our capacity to shunt people into the realms of alien otherness – 'not like us' – is one of the shadowier sides of human nature. And it often comes dressed in seductive, righteous language. It is not just on the grand stage of national and international conflicts where this darkness (masked as light) plays itself out. Its scariness is in its very ordinariness, its occurrence in everyday life among ordinary people. It doesn't happen here? But witness the nasty racist votes in the last election, in towns like Burnley and Oldham; the mob (with no sense of irony) baying for the blood of Jamie Bulger's killers; the endless undercurrent in healthcare institutions of the abuse of patients, especially the old and the mentally ill (Martin, 1984). It never goes away, and we fool ourselves if we think it does. It rests eternally at some level in every one of us, waiting.

The Jamie Bulger case – the little boy who was abducted and murdered in Liverpool by two other boys – brings many of these issues of projection into focus. We often cling to anger and hatred; they can provide a defence which if taken away would leave us to deal with our own pain. If I look deep into the recesses of my own psyche, I find lurking there what is possibly one of my deepest fears. The possibility that one of my children will die before me. I have five dear friends, all of whom have lost children under tragic, accidental circumstances. Down the years I have been filled with awe at their quiet dignity and their capacity to forgive the cause of their loss. I do not know if, faced with similar circumstances, I could find the courage to be so compassionate. I like to think I could, but . . .

So I have watched with some degree of revulsion the media spectacle at the release of the killers of Jamie Bulger. Those who howl for vengeance upon Thompson and Venables, children at the time of their crime, seem unable to see the irony of calling for their blood while damning the murder of Jamie. One TV contribution urging further retribution upon the killers cited biblical evidence in support of their cause – 'An eye for an eye' – neatly circumventing other possible quotes such as 'Vengeance is mine saith . . .' or 'Thou shalt not kill'.

Using passages from religious texts to support a cause is one of the oldest tricks in the book and it provides a rich source of contradiction and bigotry. A friend of mine who is a Jewish scholar threw up his hands in horror at the use of the 'Eye' quote to justify exposing the new identities and furthering attacks upon Thompson and Venables. He reminded me how oral Jewish tradition does not interpret this phrase in such a simplistic light; one killing does not require another. Anger and hatred are perhaps understandable in the face of such a horror as child murder, but unless there is healing and movement beyond these (see Chapter 7), the suffering is relentless, toxic and unending – feeding in ourselves the very shadow we so despise in others.

I read with astonishment the comments from one leader of the former United Kingdom Central Council for Nursing (the then governing professional body for nurses in the UK) (Rayes-Hughes, 2000), questioning whether any individual nurse should have a shadow side. We all have one! To say otherwise is to indulge in head-in-the-sand denial that feeds the possibility of this darker side of human nature expressing itself, even under the virtuous veil of caring for others. Consider the catalogue of appalling views and behaviours by a significant minority of nurses and other healthcare workers when AIDS first appeared in this country (Akinsanya & Rouse, 1991; Faugier & Hicken, 1996).

In Chapter 5 I explored the apparent positive benefits of prayer, but this too has its shadowy side, for as one study indicated (cited by Dossey, 1997a) some 5 per cent of American Christians admitted to praying for harm to come to others!

A friend of mine who would describe himself as gay was in confrontation with an eminent baroness. As to his sexuality, she said she 'would pray for him'. Look at the value judgements that lurk in that statement. He didn't want to be prayed for. He doesn't feel the need to be changed; he's happy as he is. What he wants is acceptance, not tolerance. The former is rooted in connection with another person being as whole and worthy as ourselves. The latter lurks in the nasty swamp of otherness, wearing a sweet smile while keeping its talons from view. When we create otherness, it is simply a projection on to the screen of our own lives, an outward sign that something in our divided selves is not whole, healed and integrated.

BEYOND LIGHT AND DARK?

The battle between light and dark is only one way of looking at things: that the world is a Manichean theatre of struggle between good and evil. Others may see a more complex (or simple) picture. Beyond light and dark, suggest the great mystics, lie other possibilities, a greater darkness that is also luminous – the divine light that is not dark, the darkness that has a light of its own – where all is gathered up. If this sounds paradoxical, it is, for the experience of mysticism by its very nature does not lend itself to translation into words. Yet recent studies in the emerging field of 'neurotheology' have led scientists such as Newberg et al. (2001) to suggest that the mystics were/are 'on to something'. The mystical experience teaches that 'all illustrations are inadequate and truth is beyond words', yet it offers a potential for inner transformation that enables us to be (and do) in the world differently.

The way we treat ourselves and the world is therefore dependent first of all upon some inner shift, and not upon the imposition of external rules. Karen Armstrong (1993), noting that the mystical experience is a relatively rare phenomenon, suggests that we do not have to wait for everyone to have one in order to transform, for mystics down the ages – from the Buddha to Theresa of Avila to Wayne Teasedale – have, despite the difficulties of words, been able to share their insights for the benefit of others. Dionysius the Areopagite (translated by Rolt, 1920) writes:

> The simple, absolute and immutable mysteries of divine Truth are hidden in the super-luminous darkness of that silence which revealeth the secret. For this darkness, though of deepest obscurity, is yet radiantly clear; and, though beyond touch and sight, it more than fills our unseeing minds with splendours of transcendent beauty ... We long exceedingly to dwell in this translucent darkness and through not seeing and not knowing, to see Him who is beyond both vision and knowledge – by the very fact of neither seeing Him nor knowing Him ... and here we behold that darkness beyond being, concealed under all natural light.

Thus the mystics offer us through a subtle and often perplexing veil – a glimpse of a reality beyond time and space and which brings a new perspective on the simplistic light–dark, good–evil battle. A modern mystic, Miranda Holden (2002b) is an example of this approach. Her ineffable experiences are translated into social action, grounding that which many might otherwise find bizarre or incomprehensible in practical change for the alleviation of suffering in the world.

SPIRITUAL NEUROSIS

The world is currently awash with (allegedly) enlightened beings offering us the way to God and perfect health (and the two are often promoted hand in hand). A kind of spiritual neurosis can set in as a result. This is a condition that is encountered in the face of someone who appears to be more spiritually advanced and/or enlightened than we are. Here we find ourselves awed by the mastery of the enlightened one and at the same time diminished by them – the 'We're never going to make it' feeling. The balloon of our spiritual hopes deflates in the face of those who seem so much more advanced than us; the power of their insights, the eloquence of their words, the magical manifestations – all these serve to shrink rather than encourage us. And some of these beings seem to feed on this.

I contrast this with Jesus or the Prophet or the Buddha or Guru Nanak, the founder of the Sikh faith (who, like the founders of all the great faiths, began their ministry after mystical experiences), who profoundly influenced people not just by the greatness of their presence, but also by their very ordinary humanity. For example, Jesus' words and deeds inspired and deeply moved, but he taught by a life of example, not just by telling people what to do. And it was a life that embraced the heights and depths of the human experience, including his rage in the temple, his despair at the failure of his disciples to grasp the essence of his message and his anguish and doubt as his time of trial unfolded. The mystics may reach out beyond us, but they influence our lives because they do not place themselves above us. They ask us to do nothing that is impossible, nothing that they themselves have not done. We may not all share their experience, indeed we have no need to, but they can touch our lives in such a way that we can transform the way we are in the world – a hope that grows from the fertile soil of knowing that they, like us, have walked in darkness.

I contrast this with an experience at the funeral of an acquaintance. It is not the done thing in this country to speak ill of the dead, but by the time the eulogies were over I thought, 'Crickey, I've been in the presence of a saint all these years and I didn't even know it.' Of course, she was no saint, as quiet conversations and knowledge of her life history would reveal. But I was left wondering just how healthy all this was. I have been to other funerals and wakes where the contrast could not have been starker. Yes, we spoke of their wonderful qualities, but there was a sharing of their limitations and a remembrance of their darker deeds as well, and all this was done respectfully. To do so seemed to me to honour their humanity rather than diminish it. It also takes away from us the denial that keeps us stuck in a neurotic view that we can never be as good as them. A more balanced, healthy approach to the acknowledgement of the reality of both our dark and light sides liberates us from the cage of being impossibly perfect. Setting someone upon a pedestal sets us up for disappointment in ourselves and denies the essence of what made the other person such a joyous human presence to have around.

SPIRITUAL WORK IS NO PLACE FOR SISSIES

In contrast to much of the New Age confection, which tends to be marketed as if a quick workshop here or a reading from a book there obtains instant light and bliss, all the evidence points to the reality that spiritual work is tough work. In fact, I would go so far as to say that any teacher who tells you it can all be so easy is best avoided. All teachers, great and small, alive or dead, who are or have been worth their salt, have a track record of reminding us to expect hard, often painful work. Gregory of Nyasa (translated by Roth, 1993) talks of the 'consuming fire' needed to burn off what in modern terms we would call the ego's attachments and illusions. Therapists like Frances Vaughan (1995) today write of facing the 'shadow' in order to see through the spiritual illusions of the awakening soul. The modern-day psychospiritual work *A Course in Miracles* (Anon., 1975) points out the suffering we can encounter when all the illusions of this world, of this reality, are falling away, and notes:

> 'Men have died on seeing this, because they saw no way except the pathways offered by the world. And learning they led nowhere, lost their hope. And yet this was a time when they could have learned their greatest lesson. All must reach this point and go beyond it.'

At some point in our spiritual awakening we feel the full impact of this stripping-away of notions of self. To become nothing can be deeply disturbing, so it is not surprising that many back off. 'Sometimes it is safer to be in chains than to be free' (Kafka, 1916). But all the great spiritual teachers assert that becoming nothing, no-thing, is the price of becoming everything. TS Eliot (1944)writes of 'a condition of complete simplicity, costing not less than everything'. A saying attributed to Mohammed adds: 'God has seventy thousand veils of light and darkness. If He removed them, the brilliance of His face would burn up all that met His look.' Little wonder then that spiritual practice requires the support of wise friends and counsellors, disciplined practice and attention, and reflection and silence as part of a safe approach (see also Chapters 8 and 24) if we are not to fall into madness or despair! But there is hope, as Eliot reminds us, for in the end the 'fire and the rose' become one – our restless soul, burnished of its illusions in the divine fire is reunited with its source.

AFTER THE DARK NIGHT OF THE SOUL

A healthy, deepening spiritual practice brings us to a different landscape. In fact words like 'after' or 'brings us' are misleading – for as the journey comes to a close there is a realisation that there was no journey – it just felt like it at the

time! There is just here and now, where we have always been, but viewed from
a different vantage point. There was no 'there' to get to in the first place – that
is part of the learning. And here we also see the grand illusion of the battle
between light and dark. For wholeness embraces both and takes us beyond
either, into the luminous darkness of which Dionysius speaks so eloquently.
Assaulted by Satan or the mara (in Buddhism) or the nafs (Sufism), however the
dark forces are perceived, we learn that there is no battle, for to fight the darkness is to give it strength. The qualities of being with the darkness are
paradoxical once more – relating to surrender, acceptance and acknowledgement rather than violent defence. Jesus, in his temptation by Satan, did not seek
to destroy his tempter but simply told him to get behind him. He did not fight
him or seek to use superior force against him; instead he acknowledged his
existence but refused to cooperate with him. In modern-day terms, we might
equate this with our struggle with the attachments and illusions of the ego.

Ibn Al-'Arabi reminds us that 'Then we take it back to Ourselves easily, only
because it is His shadow, since from him it is manifest and to Him the whole
manifestation returns, for the shadow is none other than He' (translated by
Austin, 1980). This notion that our personal shadow and the shadow that
is transpersonal are both of divine or cosmic origin is startling to many –
especially those who see the divine only as light in permanent opposition to
the dark. It appears to be not that simple. The celebrated German composer
Stockhausen was pilloried in the media recently when he said that he saw a
'kind of beauty' in the events of 11 September 2001 (9/11). Difficult as that may
be to comprehend, it concurs with what mystics, ancient and modern, have to
say – that beyond the events of the time and space of this reality, that which we
perceive as horror is only partially so. In a different state of reality, all such suffering that we perceive here is gathered up and transformed into that holy dark
luminosity. For God or Ultimate Reality is always beyond the reach of words
or definition – 'neti, neti' as is said in the Hindu tradition – not this, not that.

Many of us have places in our homes for those things that remind us of the
sacred – perhaps an area set aside as an altar, an icon or other religious object.
It is easy to recall the Divine, the Absolute, when we gaze upon the face of the
Buddha or Jesus, or reflect upon some words in a holy book, or turn to a picture of some special sacred place. Can we do the same if, in that same place, we
keep pictures of the ruins of 9/11, of some violent despot in a far-off country,
or some local convicted child molester?

HUNGER FOR LIGHT

Having mentioned the child molester, let's examine finally some of the shadows and projections at work there among and on these, perhaps the ultimate,

bêtes noires of our culture. Paedophiles are the villains that everybody loves to hate. Recent police enquiries and high-profile cases have flooded our media with murderous invective. Our newspapers are replete with potted psychology about adults (mainly, but not exclusively men) who want sex with children. The usual theories are banded about: it's not about sex, it's about power; it's by people who are inadequate with adult relationships seeking children; it's because the paedophile has low self-esteem.

The current frenzy and demonising of paedophiles is stifling debate and paradoxically probably increasing risk. Anyone struggling with the inner shadow of attraction to children is hardly likely to come forward for help. So they keep it bottled up until some day they pop. An alternative – a culture that permits a non-hostile dialogue on the theme, so that those at risk can seek help and effective treatment – seems hopelessly idealistic. Aye, there's the rub. To understand so that we can help and prevent, we need to hear more from paedophiles, not less. Only then can we engage understanding and make practical solutions – turning shadow into light.

As a father and now grandfather, what I have learned of paedophilia repels me. Yet all the great spiritual traditions down the ages ask me to do the opposite – for the shadow side of humanity is not reduced by pushing it away or by denial, but by embracing it with compassion and understanding that can transform darkness into light. This is a tough one, and even tougher for adults to explore with humility some of their own feelings about children. Many uncertainties lurk in our psyches that dare not speak their names.

My own childhood was rather limiting. Hugs and expressions of affection were so rare that I can remember with great clarity the few that did happen, mainly, as I wrote at the start of this chapter, at times of illness or crisis. That's not to say the love was not there; rather, no one made much of a song and dance about it. My own struggles later in life might have been different had this not been so and I deliberately set out to break the chain in terms of my interaction with my own children. We're a huggy and demonstrative family, certainly by comparison to the one I grew up in, and I believe healthier for it.

Children are immensely attractive. They draw us to them (the Darwinists would argue that this is a simple survival strategy: attention = survival) like moths to a lamp. They are charming, seductive, attention-demanding. When my children were born I just didn't want to let go of them. It's almost like you want to absorb them into yourself. Children seem to possess a light of their own and we naturally want to be around that light, to nurture and protect it. So what goes wrong with the paedophile? I think that for some people this desire to embrace and care gets distorted. A secure, fairly well-rounded adult will have developed clear boundaries around love and attraction. Consciously or unconsciously, we know when we slip across those boundaries, what is right and wrong. The adult love for a child can have intense holding and connected qualities to it – a child needs love as much as mother's milk. I wonder if some adults just can't get the feelings right and this powerful embracing quality of an adult's love for a child slips across the barrier into Eros – loving feelings get contaminated by an erotic, sexual charge normally reserved for adults. The paedophile doesn't know how to handle these mixed and distorted feelings; in fact, because they are so naturally intermingled within him, he probably doesn't see them as 'wrong' at all.

When the adult desires and covets rather than seeks to nurture the light in the child, then abuse follows. Protection is replaced by possession; lust is manifested instead of love. Children, uncluttered by ego, can seem to shine so very brightly that some adults who are not at home in themselves and their own light, and perhaps the light that rests in a deeper realm of being, may be drawn wrongly towards it. The logical conclusion is this. The 'flog 'em, castrate 'em, lock 'em up and throw away the key' model doesn't seem to work. Paedophiles will continue to be born and will continue to act out their tendencies. Psychiatric approaches seem to have yet to develop a cure, and campaigns for greater awareness, understanding and effective treatment (such as the UK and Irish organisation 'Stop it Now') struggle in the face of entrenched unbending hostility.

Is a spiritual approach a yet-unexplored option? Bringing such adults back into the light that rests within themselves and beyond themselves may be a solution. It may not only diminish the paedophiles' intentions to seek it in children, but may even help them to become more whole human beings with an adult-orientated erotic charge as a result. Perhaps the paedophile at their core does not feel whole and 'We feel separate from God or Reality' when we 'feel that we are not whole and not complete; therefore, we must take something from somebody else to get that missing completeness' (Caplan, 1999).

Our efforts to control the problem have failed and will continue to do so. Nurses, doctors and other healthcare staff are often the ones – on paediatric units and in prisons – left to pick up the broken pieces. A more imaginative dialogue and exploration of options are needed than we have had hitherto, although sadly there seem to be few signs that we are individually or collectively ready for it. Some shadows are just too deep it seems for us yet to fully enter.

My mother exposed me to chicken pox and measles so that my body could integrate them in some way, thereby becoming immune to them. Is it possible for most of us to stretch that principle to the shadow in ourselves and beyond? Are we somehow healthier and more whole when we seek to understand the darkness and embrace it for what it is – a part of all that is, waiting for light, wholeness and integration as well?

CHAPTER 14

ON THE EXISTENTIAL EDGE –
WHEN THINGS FALL APART

> *Dark and cold we may be,*
> *but this is no winter now.*
> *The frozen misery of centuries breaks,*
> *cracks,*
> *begins to move.*
> *The thunder is the thunder of floes,*
> *the thaw, the flood, the upstart spring.*
> *Thank God our time is now*
> *when wrong comes up to face us everywhere*
> *never to leave us till we take*
> *the longest stride stride of soul*
> *man ever took.*
>
> A Sleep of Prisoners, Christopher Fry (1951)

STRUCTURE

With a few countries excepted (not least my europhobically inclined home-
land), most of Europe has slipped quietly through a momentous decision – the
unification of a currency across 300 million people and many languages and
cultures, and an expansion with the addition of 11 more countries. This restructuring of a huge economy and the expansion of governance have gone better
than most have expected, and herald a gradual emergence of a unified economic, if not political, European structure.

Structure is important to us, but is also a paradox. Wherever it is created,
such as a religion, it provides a safe container for so many activities, a womb to
birth our own identities and ideas. But it may also constrain us; in keeping us
safe it may also deny us our freedom to develop, explore and grow, and even to
leave it behind, outgrown. This inherent tension is present in all structures –
social, intellectual, physical. Through long processes of preparation, it may be

possible that two structures, two 'separatenesses' such as philosophies, cultures or people can safely come together, such as I suggest in discussing healing 'union' in Chapter 18.

After the terrorist attacks in the US on 11 September 2001, that infamous date, which has now taken on iconic status (as 9/11), I determined to test some structures, not least my own inner reservations about flying when everyone else seemed determined to stay on the ground. Every one of us had our own response to that terrible event, reminding us perhaps that we live and work always on the existential edge. In an instant the solid landscape of normal orderly life can meet a precipice. Healthcare staff peer down with patients into an abyss of uncertainty when illness and injury strike. Our whole view of who we are and why we are here stares back at us. If we have never pondered those questions before, the shaking of our existential certainty may thrust us into them now.

I went to Spain, in small part to deny the post-terror paranoia, but primarily to fulfil a long-cherished wish to take someone I love to see some of the finest 'spirited' places that Europe has to offer. Spain is now thoroughly European and culturally dominated by Christianity, but it was not always so. Until the fifteenth century it was an Islamic state. Islam at that time was closer to Paris or London than it was to Mecca, and it was an Islam that was a world away from that which we so often see portrayed in the media today. Prosperous, tolerant and cultured by the standards of the time, 'Moorish' Spain saw a blossoming of inter-religious cohabitation where Judaism, Christianity and Islam flourished alongside each other. Huge advances emerged, primarily from this liberal Arabic school in medicine, chemistry, physics, philosophy and art. The great Jewish philosopher Maimonides (1135-1204) was safe enough here to produce his influential *Guide for the Perplexed* (Maimonides, translated by Rabin, 1952) – one of the great, if not the greatest, texts of Jewish thinking to emerge from the Middle Ages. His house still stands in Cordoba today, as do both the biggest mosque ever to be built outside Mecca and a fine baroque cathedral – and hereby hangs my tale.

WHEN THINGS JUST DON'T FIT

Maimonides' house has been lovingly restored. It is small and hushed, even with a murmur of tourists passing through. The walls hold biblical scripts in Hebrew. The place has a special quality to it; one might call it sacred.

The city of Cordoba was one of the last to fall to the Catholic Spanish forces, egged on by papal decree to eradicate Islam from the European continent. Soon after, a rich inheritance was swept aside in a steady tide of (often violent) repression as Spain was thoroughly Christianised. Yet today one can still walk the few yards between Maimonides' home, the mosque and the cathedral. In the aftermath of 9/11 I found much symbolism here for the root causes of that horror. The house of Maimonides fell into disrepair as the Jews were expelled from Spain. The building of the cathedral at its centre fractured the mosque, with its vast columns and perfect symmetry. It gives some idea of its scale that a cathedral could be built *within* it.

And here we see the jarring of structure. Three totally different worldviews – Judaism, Islam and Christianity – yet with so much in common, had clashed as one tried to impose its will upon the others. The architecture is supremely symbolic of this event. The merged mosque and cathedral are now a ghastly conglomeration of styles; you can watch people twisting and turning under the arches to find a vantage point that will allow them to appreciate the two styles separately. Together, they are just not compatible. Even Charles V (who had given his unthinking permission for the building of the church) was dismayed when he first saw the end result. 'You have built here what you or anyone might have built anywhere else,' he said, 'but you have destroyed what was unique in the world' (Wheaton, 1987). The architecture of this city is a metaphor for what can go disastrously wrong when one worldview seeks to impose itself upon another. The violent imagery of clashing architectures mirrors different schools of thought and belief systems, which having lost the capacity to connect with one another (losing the 'centre' of their common ground, which helped them live together amicably – a shared history, landscape, religious foundations and humanity), collapse into ignorance and destruction. Two ancient and sacred buildings have been merged in Cordoba, but the result is forced – two structures together destined forever to be apart.

The history of Spain has shown that three different religions can live amicably and prosperously together. Right relationship on this scale is founded on deep understanding and respect for each other's ways of being in the world. It seems to be a high-wire act. Human history is littered with tribalism and the capacity to create 'others' of near neighbours, as I suggested in Chapter 13. This new century sees country after country immersed in or slipping towards barbarism. A returning Jesus, Abraham, Buddha or Mohammed might well be forgiven for thinking that they wasted their time. Yet there is hope and it lies not only in the grand scheme of things but also seeded in the way each one of us conducts our own lives.

WE LIVE ALWAYS ON THE EXISTENTIAL EDGE

The solid landscape of normal orderly life meets a precipice. Those who work with the sick peer down with them into the abyss of uncertainty when illness and injury strike. The victims of terror, those dear to them and those beyond, stare over the same precipice when normal life – our buildings, our work, our hopes and expectations – are broken beneath us. Things fall apart when our centre can no longer hold, as the poet WB Yeats (in Webb, 1991) reminds us.

Tragedy on a grander scale does more than shake our individual paradigms – our collective worldview can be shaken into a new form. Such an event was 9/11, already hailed as 'the day that changed the world' in many media headlines at the time. Whether with hindsight this will prove to be so remains to be seen. There is evidence that a significant cultural shift, in the Western world at least, is under way: people are turning away from materialistic lifestyles towards global, personal and spiritual wellbeing and concerns (Ray, 1996; Thomas, 1999). 'Ground Zero' may have accelerated this – a reminder 'of how fragile life is' and causing people to ask themselves, 'If I were facing death could I say that I have done everything I wanted?' (Pierpoint, 2001). Nobody ever died wishing they had spent more time at the office!

However, for others 'The response has been to go out and indulge themselves quite literally as if there were no tomorrow. A new car. New designer clothes. Even consumption of illegal drugs is up' (Pierpoint, 2001). Other signs have not been optimistic. Two American televangelists were quick to condemn the events as punishment for America's tolerance of abortion, homosexuality, divorce – not noticing the irony that such views would make them comfortable bedfellows with their Islamic fundamentalist counterparts! The polarising of people into good and evil, creating tribes of 'us' and 'them', allowed the warlike bandwagon to roll on. Gandhi, Luther King and others have shown the power of compassion and non-violence, but our resort to war exposes how far we have yet to evolve cultures able to resolve conflict peacefully. Other ways, slower and more patient, lack the telegenic drama of war rhetoric and smart bombs and do not feed the hunger for vengeance. Retaliation may be a right, but it is a right that can be renounced.

We may have been changed by 9/11, for it was a spiritual crisis in every sense – challenging so many people to reflect upon the meaning and purpose of their lives and how to live them, and forcing us to confront many established views about each other and our belief systems. It is no coincidence that the fastest selling book after 9/11 was the Qur'an. This was not to feed some renewed religious fervour, but because huge numbers of people wanted to know more about a faith of which they knew little and which perplexed them in its capacity to nurture suicidal assassins.

What many will have learned is that this is not an Islamic problem. It happens to focus on Islam right now because of all kinds of political, national, religious and economic factors. But, there but for the grace of God go . . . History is replete with the capacity of all faiths to generate the basest of human emotions as well as the most noble. The fundamentalist outlook lurks in the nest of many faiths, waiting to be fed and nurtured into some monstrous manifestation. In the twentieth century it took on a peculiarly bellicose mantle — 'a reaction against the scientific and the secular' (Armstrong, 2001). It is less of a clash between nation states of one faith, more a clash within faiths and nations, the liberal and the authoritarian, the religious and the secular. A deep malaise, a spiritual sickness, lies at the centre of modern conflict that is intricate and complex in its causes, stark and brutal in its effects.

BEING THE PEACE WE SEEK

In the face of atrocity on such a scale, we could be forgiven for feeling overwhelmed and hopeless. We cannot rely just upon the great and good to resolve matters. For societies to work together, the solutions lie in each one of us. Healthcare workers do not live in isolation. We and those we serve may have been changed by 9/11 — were you? We *are* society and the values we hold, and practices we pursue influence the greater whole. Holding prayerful intentions for peace and healing *does* have an impact, as the studies on prayer and intention in Chapter 5 indicate. How we deal with our own anger and grief over such an event has an impact beyond ourselves, permeating all our relationships, both personal and professional.

Nurses, doctors and other carers have a track record of 'containerising' things, a delusion that by boxing up 'our stuff' we can just carry on caring. Don't you believe it! We are not boxes, we are sieves full of holes that consciously or unconsciously reveal to others in all sorts of ways just where we are with ourselves. From our hands and our mouths in every interaction with patients, we reveal ourselves. If we accept notions of the holistic universe (be we mystics or quantum physicists), then the whole is affected by its parts. Wanting peace and the relief of suffering starts within ourselves, by being the peace we seek, by being in the world in ways that relieve suffering — both our own and others.

Evil never comes out of good, but good can come out of evil. So many shibboleths and holy cows have had to be confronted since 9/11 — the use and abuses of power, the nature of fundamentalism, religious stereotypes and libertarian ideals. We see the paradox of faith, a comfort to the bereaved and dying but fuel to the deathwish of the assassin. Seeing danger, perhaps we can discover ways to avoid it. 'The demons of Western culture and Islam are now out in the open' (Beddington-Behrens, 2001), providing an opportunity amongst the suffering to confront them.

Out of the shadow we saw the best of human beings. A victim's wife begging a president not to go to war and create more widows. Forlorn nurses and doctors waiting for patients who never came. Firemen entering a building they must have known was doomed. And, above all, those answerphone-sealed calls from myriad mobiles – 'I love you'. Even unto death, and perhaps beyond, love endured unmoved, a bastion against all that murder and mayhem in their futility could cast against it. Love is the structure that holds our centre together; it *is* the centre. Without it, all beliefs, all systems, all relationships fall apart.

CHAPTER 15
RECLAIMING THE CRONE

Looking into the mirror I spotted
a single strand of grey hair
and plucked it out. 'I'm easy game alone,'
it said, 'but what do you plan
to do with my troops close behind me?'

Yehuda Halevi (translated by Levin, 2002)

BEFORE THE PARTY

To an Englishman rooted in the hard winters of the North, the climate of California is a grand seduction. I immersed myself in the delights of the hot tub under warm early morning sunshine and watched a solitary deer at the bottom of the garden watching me watching her. Neither of us gave way, until the Pleasant Valley Cleansing Company of Walnut Creek crushed the silence with the rattle of wheelie bins and the dull grind of the hoisting of rubbish into the truck. When I looked back, she was gone.

An old woman emerged from her porch, bowed under the weight of ragged newspapers, and dumped them near the truck. The workmen were young; the woman had the kind of deep craggy wrinkles that are folded into the face by hard sun over many years, and a few moments of flirtatious banter followed before she melted back into the shadows of her house. The young men laughed their way to the next street.

For some reason this little scene stuck in my mind for the rest of the day as we prepared the house for a grand party – a celebration of my companion's 70 years' walking this earth. People came and went, we sang songs, read poems, played music and probably ate and drank more than was good for us. The culmination was a rebirthing ceremony with joyous clapping and singing to a Navajo chant. We celebrated her arrival into cronedom at 70 years, the passing

point into revered old age where all the accumulated wisdom could take on a
new purpose in the service of others.

Not a few people at the party winced at the word 'crone', for it has come
to be a pejorative term in our culture. The dictionary (Allen, 1990) defines a
crone as a 'withered old woman' and points out that the origins lie in the Old
Norse and early French word *carogne*, meaning carrion. Other words for old
women tend to have negative connotations, too, reinforced by several thousand
years of patriarchy – hags, wicked witches and evil stepmothers pepper our language and mythology, and only the rare fairy godmother escapes. Old men,
however, get off much more lightly with more positive associations, be they
sages, elder statesmen or powerful business magnates (often with much younger
brides in tow). In previous chapters I have explored the need to enter the shadow in all its forms in the search for integration. Our individual and collective
response, the casting of the shadow over the older woman, seems to be a territory worth exploring a little more.

BRINGING BACK THE FEMININE

Twenty years ago I had the pleasure of befriending a 70-year-old woman who
became something of a celebrity in the UK. Jane Saxby for a while was a star
on the conference circuit, especially those associated with the care of older
people, not least because she was brave enough to be the woman who was willing to talk about sex (Saxby, 1983a). But she was a rare phenomenon at the
time. Perhaps things are changing, but if so the pace is slow.

Achterberg (1990) and Cope (1998) graphically illustrate the systematic
destruction of women's power and influence over thousands of years. Masculine gods and power worldviews took over much of the world, yet modern
health care cries out for a restoration of the feminine perspective and sees its
manifestation perhaps in the rise of the complementary therapies, with their
emphasis on healing, nurturing, empowerment and comfort. A tide is flowing
that the best efforts of the (usually male) sceptics and scientists are unable to
stem. Women seem to be in the majority flowing with this tide, both as users
and providers of complementary care, yet the tide is not drowning modern
medicine – rather seeking to wash upon its shores and merge with it. An
increasing willingness is being shown to integrate orthodox and complementary approaches to health and healing (Foundation of Integrated Health,
2003), and that willingness is coming from both sides. Achterberg (1990) sees
this process as crucial:

> *The emergence of women whose consciousness blends with the ancient themes of healing
> is the single most promising event in health care, for the lack of a feminine point of view*

is the most abject omission in modern institutions and at the heart of the problems in modern medicine. The manifestation of feminine values in medicine is critical for the health of the planet.

The full manifestation of the feminine in modern health care has yet to be achieved and it is intimately bound up with the possibility of reasserting the value of the crone as the wise old woman, for without her the feminine in all its aspects is incomplete. It is perhaps against the crone that the bastions of masculinity hold most firm, for she represents the power and wisdom that can only come with the advance of years. The hostility to powerful women may explain some of the negativity to female spiritual teachers or their disappearance off the stage in the stories of the emergence of the great religions. In so many religious traditions, women barely get a look-in and their contribution has often been edited out of their history. Where women do get a role, it is often quite clear that it is a secondary one to men. The recent furore in the Church of England over the ordination of women is still a deep wound for many in the Church, and many parishioners have refused to accept a woman priest. Other faiths, too, have their 'women problems' – the C of E is not the only one to have difficulty.

While women are excluded, the feminine is also held apart; yet in a holy (wholy, holistic) enterprise, where the Divine, Ultimate Reality, the Absolute is invariably described as 'One' – then separation, exclusion, dualism in any form is surely contrary to this principle. The separatist, denialist approach may fuel the dismissal of old women especially, and this requires a 'respiriting' of ageing if the ageing process for all of us is to become healthy.

Older women themselves may be seduced by all the social messages of their worthlessness or ugliness, even though there are signs, especially in the feminist literature and the arts, that this is being challenged. Older women, reveals Jane Saxby (1983b), are hardly likely to share their strengths with others when they themselves may not value or be aware of them, or fear the effects if they 'come out'. 'They do not expect to be portrayed as ridiculous, ugly, obscene and unnatural and so will not reveal their precious and private memories unless assured of honour and dignity.'

THE SCARY WOMAN

It is something of a truism that, if we fear something, the way to deal with it is to make it an object of ridicule or diminish its power by diminishing its importance. In discussions with male friends I have often raised the topic of what it is they/we fear most in the world. The expected topics are raised – disease, loss of job, death of self or a loved one, extreme pain and many others. Lurking in the background unacknowledged and indeed dismissed, if suggested, is the fear of the feminine. I have often felt that the most terrifying thing a man can encounter is the feminine. It is one of the best-kept secrets of men. Behind all the posturing, bravado, control and manifestation of masculine power lies the deeply hidden knowledge (so deep that some of us men dare not even believe that it is there) that the feminine, and by extension women, terrify us.

This knowledge lies at the bottom of our psyche, lurking like a shark in the black depths, creeping out to attack us like a thief in the night, hanging around the corners of the shadows of our minds, waiting to consume us just when we think we have got it all sorted. For thousands of years we (men) have successfully relegated the fear of the feminine to the backwaters of our consciousness. By keeping women firmly in their place, and destroying or controlling any significant role or power they have in our culture, the feminine was also kept tightly under wraps. The (relatively) few powerful women in recent history, from Elizabeth I to Margaret Thatcher, were only allowed to be so because they portrayed strong masculine attributes. In Christianity, the Church has historically had real problems with the most powerful woman of them all: Mary, the mother of Jesus. Her cult has often been repressed and she has been relegated to a curiously safe, submissive and sexless role (it is rarely mentioned that Jesus had other siblings). Jung (1961), however, has remarked that the elevation of Mary to divine status by the Catholic Church in the twentieth century was one of that century's most significant cultural and spiritual acts. Woman and the feminine were being reintegrated with God, and Jung believed that this will play itself out in many unforeseen ways in the future, which will be of profound significance.

Despite Shekinah, the feminine creative aspect of the divine in Judaism, Sophia, the feminine power of wisdom, the Virgin Mary, the Buddhist Tara or the significant role played by the Prophet's first, rich, older and powerful wife in Islam, it is largely the men who have made all the running in the great faiths of recent years. The feminine deity, if acknowledged at all (bearing in mind that most early faiths seem to have been goddess-orientated), has been carefully subsumed under the power of the male god. Paradoxically, many of the great religious figures such as Jesus and the Buddha were men who exhibited strong feminine qualities of kindness, inclusiveness, love and compassion. Yet, if the feminine is to be integrated into health care, then by extension it must be integrated into our belief systems. And to do that the men are going to have to do a lot more work integrating the feminine in themselves.

This is a call for men not just to adopt the caring-sharing values of the 'New Man' (or take off in search of the 'wild man' inside in an effort to re-clarify and re-assert his masculinity (Bly, 1990)), but also to seek out and explore and integrate their own femininity. For that is holism, that is healing: the balance of opposing and yet complementary forces within the one, the yin and yang of

Daoism in eternal harmonious dance with each other, representing as they do the same balance of forces in the cosmos. As above, so below. All spiritual paths invite us towards wholeness and emergence into the Divine, the One, the Absolute; yet a man who does not bring the feminine and the masculine into balance within him is not complete. Does an incomplete man get to God?

But this is scary stuff, for the feminine represents all men's deepest fears. In Hinduism, for example, the goddess Kali, the ultimate creative and destructive force, is at once terrifying and awesome. She holds in herself the power to create new life, a rich symbol of procreation, but also the gate of death, for death and birth are inextricably bound in the cycle of life. Try as he might, man cannot deny that he emerges from mysterious woman and back into that dark mystery he must return. All his individuality, his power, his achievements must come to naught, for the same valley of death awaits us all.

For generations men have controlled women and by extension the feminine. But the victory has always been transitory, for Kali's sword awaits us all at the end. The old woman, the crone, who has passed beyond the dictates of what men have decided is attractive, coupled with her deep and hidden well of wisdom, stands before men as a final insult to what they thought was their power.

HOPE

The rebirthing of the crone may be a sign for optimism, for 'women who join together with each other to deny the male God who cursed their sex and to reject his demands for obedience, praise, service and money automatically free themselves from one of the most potent psychological traps men ever set for them'. Furthermore, men's fear of the power of the crone is the chink in their armour that will let in the challenge to men's 'ego trips, war toys and money games' (Walker, 1985).

I am blessed to have not a few crones in my circle and one in particular who has been at many levels my own personal Kali. It makes for a fiery relationship, but it is a fire that burnishes the soul and prepares me ever more for the journey Home. But beyond the personal impact, the rise of the crone's power once more would infiltrate every level of our culture and bring back into balance those extremes, which not only undermine the best intentions of our health-care system, but also threaten the very existence of the planet itself. In our culture, growing old is increasingly seen as a 'problem' for society. Faced with an ageing population, it desperately needs positive role models of ageing and dependency if we are to counter these trends (see also Chapter 22). If 'doing' gets more difficult for all kinds of reasons as we get older, there is still the potential of 'being' – the capacity, even in the face of disadvantage or disability, to radiate our wisdom, our experience, our loving presence with others. I have met many older people who fall into that category of 'being', offering as much, if not more, than if they were 'doing'. Accepting such role models would have immense benefits to a culture that remains ageist and misogynist on many levels. It is the added layer of misogyny that makes it doubly important for us to re-evaluate the crone.

Women are not exclusively feminine and men are not exclusively masculine. The power of the crone stands available to us to bring both into a new and healing harmony for 'both genders need a well-differentiated masculine as well as well-differentiated feminine' if we are to escape the 'structures of patriarchy' that have so 'profoundly wounded both' (Woodman & Dickson, 1996).

AFTER THE PARTY

I sat alone on the grassy bank. It was a clear night and the moon, so often a symbol of the feminine, was full and brilliant. It seemed appropriate to sit beneath it at the end of a joyous celebration, a public acknowledgement of a woman not in decline, or ugly or useless, but a woman coming into her own. Men and women have much to do together to forge an appreciation of age as power. The wise man, the sage, has suffered less from ageism than the woman. The wisdom that lies in the crone is waiting for its time once more, another step towards integration, 'and so the time comes when all the people of the earth can bring their gifts to the fire and look into each other's faces unafraid' (Starhawk, cited in Anderson, 1996).

The power inherent in ageing is not whole if its feminine side is not ranked as equal alongside it. To be otherwise creates a world out of balance. An ageing that is not whole is an age that is not whole.

CHAPTER 16

DO WINTER BUFFALO DREAM OF SUMMER MEADOWS?

We perceive some doings as good
and some as evil,
but our Lord
does not perceive them so.
For just as everything that exists
in nature
is created by God,
so also is everything that is done
God's own doing.
There is no doer but God.

Julian of Norwich (translated by Doyle, 1983)

YELLOWSTONE

Like an old shirt worn too long, a national park at the end of the season has that overly lived-in look, the tracks too worn, the grassland tired and blanched, the forest hanging damp in the morning chill, waiting for the crisp bite of frost. An early snow completes the evacuation of the tourists, and car parks and camping stations sit vacant and silent under steel-grey clouds. The silence runs deep, the kind of silence that follows long-gone crowds; the excited voices of children and the yelps of dogs but a ghostly echo. When the vulgar raven calls, he is subdued. Even he, the solitary resident of the empty picnic shelter, seems to call more to reassure himself that he is still there. No raucous belch to see off a rival or to demand the contents of a left-over packed lunch. In Yellowstone, Wyoming, the rangers seem happy to be dropping those big gates to close the roads, and smile a particular smile kept reserved for just those moments when autumn slips into winter. No more the weary late-season rictus grin for the millionth Winnebago. The face can drop, the holidaymakers gone; this is the smile of 'no entry', of anticipation of quiet days, of the return to peace.

We made it through for the last run up the main road before the rangers declared the park a no-go area. Bereft of the tourist gangs, the park put on a special evening show of elk, coyote and buffalo. The buffalo (more accurately, bison), with their massive shoulders and matted brown hides, have the look of beasts that are used to being looked at. Their sullen hunched air, indifferent to the click of cameras or the swerve of cars to catch a glimpse, continued as they lumbered from trees to plain. Numbed by the countless intrusive pointings and cacklings of excited humans, they seem quite simply to have become oblivious to our existence. Crowds or no crowds, it makes no difference. We are un-registered on their awareness.

The deepening cold of winter in Yellowstone sinks deep into you. Altitude and unseasonal snow conspire to produce a bone-cold chill. I dreamed of piping hot food and a roaring fire to relieve my encroaching discomfort. The buffalo passed us by, walking with steaming nostrils into winter deprivation. Do visions of the wild flowers of summer and sweet meadow grass run through their heads while they stand with their backs to ice-clad mountains?

SUFFERING IS GRACE

My musings on animals – about their awareness and actual or potential suffering – reinforced my long-held view that they are probably Zen Buddhists. It is difficult to know exactly what is going on in the consciousness of a non-human, but on the surface at least they appear to have an in-bred capacity for living in the moment. There is a story of a journalist attending the workshop of a Zen master. Struggling to understand the essential concepts of Zen and desperately needing some clarity for his report, he ensured he sat next to the master during lunch.

'Can you define for me what Zen is really all about?' the journalist enquired.

'Eat' said the master.

'But what exactly is it?' he pressed.

'Eat' said the master.

'Surely you can give some useful explanatory quotes for my journal?'

'Eat' said the master.

Exasperated, the journalist went to the bar and ordered a stiff gin and tonic.

Zen-like, most animals just seem to be attending to what they are doing at the time. They rarely, if ever, give the impression that their minds are elsewhere. Watching those buffalo, there was no indication that they were thinking 'Snow's here, winter's on its way and I might die or get attacked by wolves.' They were simply busy being buffalo, walking when they were walking, drinking when they were drinking, eating when they were eating – just in the moment without apparent fears for present or future.

Human beings seem to find it a much tougher prospect to stay in the moment. We can not only be stuck in the pain and suffering we experience in the present, but also embellish it with memories of what has been, or exacerbate it with anguish about what might be. 'Suffering is,' said the Buddha, and the human experience explores every countless facet of it. We cannot *not* suffer.

In the face of suffering, be it our own or others', it seems we have a number of options. We can, for example, drown it in the pursuit of pleasure or distraction that fills every moment – work, sex, drugs, alcohol, shopping, television. We can surrender into the 'unyielding despair' that Russel (cited in Schumacher (1977) believes is the only option if we feel that 'this is all there is', faced with a seemingly pointless universe, which may be no more than a 'random collocation of atoms'. Or we may look at suffering as purposeful. Ram Dass (2000), his experience and teachings reinforced by his stroke several years ago, echoes the work of many great spiritual teachers both past and present – that suffering is purposeful, most specifically in being the grist for the mill, the rough grit to polish away the ego so that the soul can (re)unite with the divine. Faced with the reality of serious illness or the death of a loved one, to see 'suffering as grace', as a blessing to free us from the traps of the ego, can be a very tall order indeed if we have not had the spiritual practice to bring us to this point.

Sitting here with my (reasonably) healthy if slightly overweight body, it is relatively easy to accept the theory of suffering as grace – an opportunity, and sometimes harsh teacher, to help me unpick the illusions of my ego self and come ever more deeply into an awareness of who I really am and why I am here. I can look back now upon the many periods of often deep distress in my life and see that out of the pain came healing and transformation – usually, but not always, in the long term. This is the true nature of what *A Course in Miracles* (Anon., 1975) calls 'the Forgiveness' – not a mere letting-go of the 'wrongs' done to us by others, but a profound awareness that there was no 'wrong' at all, really. Thus every action, no matter how painful it may seem at the time, is chosen by our souls and is perfectly placed, exquisitely crafted to burnish away the illusion of who we think we are, in order to come to an ever-closer awareness of the true Self. The conclusion of this process, if words like 'conclusion' in this respect have any meaning at all, is often most clearly expressed in mystical and transcendent terms. The great Sufi mystic Abu Yazid Bistami sees suffering as leading to the death of self in order to see truth:

> *I gazed upon Allah with the eye of truth and said to Him: 'Who is this?' He said, 'This is neither I nor other than I. There is no God but I.' Then he changed me out of my identity into His selfhood . . . Then I communed with him with the tongue of his Face saying; 'How fares it with me with Thee?' He said, 'I am through Thee, there is no god but Thou.'* cited in Armstrong, 1993

GRACE IS JUST A DEFENCE MECHANISM!

An interesting piece of recent research looks at whether human beings are somehow innately 'wired' in our brains to connect to God (Newberg et al., 2001). Hamer's (2004) DNA studies suggest that an inclination to faith is the product of genetically determined brain chemicals. Sartre famously hoped that once God was dead (i.e. atheism through reason prevailed) then the 'God shaped hole' in our consciousness could be filled with a rational approach to solving humanity's problems (cited in Armstrong, 2000). The assumption that part of us is somehow open to God, but could be filled by something else is debatable, and Newberg and his colleagues in the emerging field of neurotheology are providing some fascinating scientific evidence. They conclude that, in effect, the religious impulse is rooted in the biology of the brain.

One interesting theory is put forward in their thinking. In a nutshell it goes something like this. As our consciousness evolved from ape to human being millennia ago we became aware of our mortality and our minuteness in the face of the vastness of the universe. Some human beings would find such a prospect so daunting that they would be inclined to nihilism or depression and therefore were more likely to die. The human beings that survived did so because they developed experiences/belief systems that gave them hope, for example of an afterlife. They were better equipped to live because they had the prospect of something 'more' than ordinary reality. Thus, in the best Darwinian tradition, they were more likely to survive and reproduce, and thus human beings are around today with brains attuned to God because our ancestors who were not just did not make it down the genetic survival chain.

It's a fascinating theory and probably meat and drink to modern-day Darwinists. It assumes there isn't really a God, that we somehow created one in order to survive this sometimes rather nasty world we must inhabit and the extreme suffering we often experience. There is, of course, a different theory. That there is a God or ultimate reality and the god-shaped hole in our consciousness was thus ordered so we could connect to a reality deeper and grander than this one. The mystics, of course, would see the former explanation as tosh, the 'this is all there is' types the latter in a similar vein. And God (whoever or however you see him/her/it) is probably laughing all the way to the gene bank!

THE GREAT CONUNDRUM

If suffering is grace, an ultimately beneficial force that enables us to reunite with the Source, then why bother to intervene to prevent or reduce it? Why take away pain from the post-operative patient? Why feed the starving? Why stop the murderer? To intervene in this process is to delay us on the path Home. Yet suffering abounds all around us and our 'natural' instinct is to seek to reduce it – it is the seedbed of countless helping occupations, the very ground of our human relationships from the time the mother suckles the child. If suffering is grace, then every tyrant in history has in fact been a great angel of mercy – despatching huge numbers of people out of this reality and on into the next. How can we make sense of this apparently senseless conundrum?

In his attempted rewriting of the Hippocratic oath, the physician Allan Butler (1968) wrote, 'We physicians shall re-emphasize as basic to our profession the rational ethical principle of minimizing suffering.' Rational and ethical it may be, but without a deeper exploration of the nature of suffering, something that the humanistic approach has tended to skirt around, then it is difficult to be sure exactly what we are being rational and ethical about. Furthermore, suffering by its very nature may not lend itself easily to clarity through reason and ethical debate.

Perhaps the answer, if there is one, lies in seeing suffering from many different perspectives and coming to rest more easily in uncertainty. First, there are the collective and interconnected aspects of suffering. If we are all ultimately part of the whole, then one person's suffering is also my suffering. In helping another I am also helping myself. When I witness the starving child and I intervene to feed that child, I not only relieve the child, I also diminish my own pain at witnessing that child in distress. I feel better when others feel better (but notice the co-dependency trap here for the caring professionals, the risk of getting caught up in superhood leading to burnout as we drown out our own needs in an effort to sort out everyone else's; see Chapter 4). At a deeper level, the relief of one person's suffering is also the relief of *the* suffering, the collective experience and presence of it. Helping and healing are mutual processes.

Second, we can examine the intention with which we approach suffering. While honestly witnessing and being party to our own agendas (see also Chapter 5 on prayer and intentionality) when we encounter the pain of others, the spiritual practice of healing work involves learning to let go of our attempts to be in control of it all. The great Christian mystic Meister Eckhart reminds us of this quality to be cultivated when he urges us to 'Examine yourself, and wherever you find yourself, then take leave of yourself. This is the best way of all' (Eckhart, translated by Davies, 1994). Taking leave of ourselves does not mean that we do not act; rather that we approach our actions with humility – being aware of our own needs and desires, watching ourselves when we are caught up in the grand drama of suffering, and setting it all to one side as we do what has to be done. 'We do nothing, and nothing is left undone' (Ram Dass & Gorman, 1990). There is doing, but it is not 'ours'.

The Hindu tradition has the Baghavad Gita as one of its deepest foundations, a mythic-religious epic on a vast scale with two main beings, Arjuna and his god-like teacher, Krishna, who guides him through the vicissitudes of life. Amidst the mayhem of the field of battle, Arjuna weeps in anguish – to fight or not to fight? He appeals for help and guidance from the Lord Krishna: 'In the dark night of my soul I feel desolation. In my self-pity I see not the way of righteousness. I am thy disciple, come to thee in supplication: be a light unto me on the path of duty' (Mascaro, 1962). Faced with the pain of suffering laid out before him, Arjuna meets the classic interior struggle of all who seek to 'do the right thing'. Krishna essentially advises him that he must choose to act. If Arjuna does something, there will be consequences. If he seemingly does nothing, there will be consequences. We cannot not participate!

LIGHT WARRIORS?

However, it is the grounding of that action on which Krishna further advises, urging Arjuna on to a deeper understanding of life and death. 'The wise grieve not for those who live; and they grieve not for those who die – for life and death shall pass away,' he says. He encourages him onward into war but reminds him to be clear in his intentions. 'Prepare for war with peace in thy soul. Be in peace in pleasure and in pain, in gain and in loss, in victory or in loss of battle. In peace there is no sin.' This peace comes from embracing a deeper reality than the Manichean battle between the forces of light and dark, for 'God is all'.

There is much talk in New Age spirituality and indeed some 'old age' spirituality of being 'light warriors'. We need to be wary of this title. It risks nudging us into reductionist and dualistic views of the world, simplistic notions of black and white, light and dark. We are the 'goodies' fighting for the light against the 'bad' dark. Indeed, the term 'light warrior' is something of a spiritual oxymoron unless it is used only in the metaphorical sense. Like the current use of 'war against terrorism', the phrase is imbued with contradiction. We do not wage war against terror, for to wage war is to create terror. We are not warriors of light, for the light does not wage war. 'War' is the tool of the shadow, the destructive force of the 'not being'. We do not wage war on darkness, for to do so is to become darkness by using the very tools that are the stuff of darkness itself.

Those of us who seek to help others need to be wary of locking ourselves into separation, into identification with roles that set us apart from the 'other' (for indeed there is no other). We can get caught up in too much righteous doing, as opposed to being with people in their suffering. Once again, this does not mean that we do not act (for we cannot not act!), rather that when we do act we do so from a place of deep surrender of our own will to The Will. Krishna again:

> In the bonds of works I am free, because in them I am free from desires. The man who
> can see this truth, in his work he finds freedom ... When work is done as sacred work,

unselfishly, with a peaceful mind, without lust or hate, with no desire for reward, then the
work is pure. Mascaro, 1962

Guidance like that of Krishna can be found in all the great spiritual traditions. It is the very essence of all those who work to relieve suffering, be we
nurses, doctors or therapists of whatever denomination. Working in and with
suffering is spiritual work, for both helper and helped, for in it we recognise
the limitations of our labels and our actions. Recognising these limitations of
established theories, practices, roles and boundaries can produce a transformation in those who work in the helping professions. We may come to an
awareness that our work is about not just doing but also being. Who we are
around people can be a relief to suffering of itself. We are all in this together.
Suffering is an opportunity for awakening both for ourselves and the other;
indeed it may be a manifestation of our experience of suffering that we recognise that there is no other. For the helper, there may be not only a gateway to
relieve suffering in the most direct and obvious ways – I will not hesitate to
halt someone throwing themselves suicidally out of the window of the psychiatric ward; would not wait to give that painkilling injection to the post-op
child; would not stop to question in fighting off the mugger attacking my
neighbour – but also an opening for spiritual awakening. Here there may be
a precious moment not only to do what I do, but also to be with the other
sensitively, carefully, in humility, to explore the deeper meaning of that suffering. In so doing we may not only help in the relief of suffering, but also coach
a subtle shift of consciousness in the sufferer about what their suffering is all
about.

The Hindu tradition holds that the consciousness we have at the moment
of death determines the path of our next lifetime and how close we get to
God. Gandhi famously turned himself to the divine even at the moment of his
assassination with his last word 'Ram' (God). His last thought was of God, and
also a teaching to the crowd: 'This too is God.' There may be some added element here about the way we may intervene in suffering. Acts of malice and
violence, especially if random and spontaneous, provide little opportunity to
make any shift of consciousness. We are simply forced to instantly deal with
what is. At a deeper, soul level we may know that 'All shall be well', but that
may be a tall order of perception when faced with the empty food bowl or the
gut-shrinking pain. But if suffering is grace, it is grace for the one called to
helping as well, for we are given blessed moments pregnant with the potential
that if we are with them in 'peaceful mind' those shifts of consciousness towards
Home might take place. Then working with suffering is truly sacred work.

CHAPTER 17

MAKING A SPECTACLE OF A MIRACLE

> All things in heaven come about in existence
> Existence comes about in non-existence . . .
> Both are one in origin
> and different only in name.
> Its unity is called the secret.
> The secret's still deeper secret
> is the gateway through which all miracles
> emerge.
>
> Tao Te Ching (Streep, 1994)

THE DEAD HAND OF SCIENCE

Many chapters in this book have discussed elements of the nature of healing and the resolution of things which are fragmented into oneness, wholeness, holiness. Spirituality is about coming to rest at Home in the oneness of things, making sense and meaning of our lives and the world. Healing, which as we have discussed is closely related to the words 'holism', 'healthy' and 'holy', is one of the building blocks of spirituality. Much modern writing and teaching, and the multitude of courses on the subject, are delineating healing as a 'therapy' (from the Greek 'therapia' – healing) – and this may be its undoing.

The modern scientific medical paradigm demands a rationale for all health-care practices, and this trend is fuelled by government-sponsored bodies such as NICE in the UK (the National Institute for Clinical Excellence) and similar organisations in other countries, which have immense influence over which therapies can and cannot be available to patients. As Abbot points out in a helpful survey of the current evidence for healing from randomised clinical trials, 'Hard evidence of effectiveness is increasingly required for therapeutic interventions' and 'Emphasising clinical efficacy and cost-effectiveness of service provision is likely to increase the pressure on therapies such as healing to expand their evidence base, preferably through randomised controlled trials' (Abbot, 2000). Monitoring the research base for a particular treatment, making a judgement on its effectiveness and then recommending whether it should or should not be used are a sweetly seductive approach. This is especially so when we have to account for the spending of public money and the protection of the public from charlatanism and quackery.

And charlatanism and quackery there are in abundance, thickly layered with added spreadings of irresponsibility and non-accountability. Leafing through the pages of any New Age journal, or come to that, much of the mainstream press, reveals a plethora of adverts for training in healing – with little evidence that users and students of such services are properly and safely vetted before-hand or effectively followed up afterwards. Anyone can call themselves a healer (despite the efforts of organisations such as the National Federation of Spiritual Healers to set standards of training and practice).

Furthermore, large numbers of healers seem hooked into a particular model whereby they assume themselves to be channels or focuses of 'healing energy' (be it divine or otherwise), which is then transmitted or applied in some way to the patient or client (Hodges & Scofield, 1995). Thus a healer–healee relationship is set up. There are serious flaws in this approach, too, which under-mine the potential for healing and feed the sceptics who wish to debunk heal-ing at any opportunity.

First of all, science currently only recognises four forms of energy – gravi-tational, electromagnetic, and strong and weak nuclear (Dossey, 1997b). To use 'energy' so randomly, as so many in the work of healing do, is to expose their practice to ridicule from the scholarly and those who prefer to keep to strict scientific discipline. It does not help the understanding or acceptance of heal-ing if such people are alienated from the discourse through sloppy con-ceptualising. Second, a healer–healee relationship is not holistic; it is reduc-tionist and dualistic. Holism, another much-abused word, is about the oneness of all things, not separation into distinct roles. Healer–healee is just the same as doctor–patient, a dualistic separation of one from another that suggests one working with or doing to another. Whichever the case, despite the almost uni-versal claims by those working in healing ways to holistic principles, to speak of healer and healee is a contradiction in terms, a therapeutic oxymoron. It is not possible to assert that 'healers' work holistically, yet follow the old medical model of setting themselves apart from the one that comes to them for help.

Such contradictions are manna from heaven to those of a sceptical persuasion. Some are sceptical for positive reasons, seeking knowledge and understanding to prevent wholesale acceptance of distorted or dangerous practices. Others are sceptical for the hell of it, determined from that deep fearful place in their psy-ches to quash anything that does not fit neatly with their particular worldview.

ORGANIC HEALTH CARE

People turn away from orthodox therapies to the complementary precisely because they are different. They offer largely comforting approaches to care, with time and attention, which are often so lacking in the intensive health care of the mainstream health systems. Western health care has developed an intensive approach to health not dissimilar to that of agriculture – maximum productivity (patient throughput) from minimal effort (least cost). Just as the public is turning away from the methods of intensive, factory-farming agriculture to more environmentally friendly and organic approaches to stock and crop rearing, so people have increasingly rejected intensive health care for more holistic approaches. The complementary therapies, with their tendency towards comfort and relaxation, self-empowerment and one-to-one attention, have ridden the crest of this wave of change. Embracing many approaches to healing, they have become the equivalent in health care to the rise in organic farming in agriculture.

However, a complementary therapy is not necessarily holistic per se, nor does the practitioner necessarily work in such a way. It is just as easy to find complementary practitioners who are as obsessed with their particular technique as any mainstream practitioner might be with their own bit of health technology. What seems to be of significance in healing is not just the technique but the quality of the relationship with the practitioner – relationships characterised by awareness, trust, mutuality, openness and, yes, love, i.e. 'right relationship'. Right relationship is a hallmark of holistic practice and it is this that may be the trigger that sets off the inherent capacity of people to heal themselves. Thus certain approaches to healing may work regardless of techniques, simply because the 'patient' believes in or has faith in the therapy and practitioner, feels good in their presence and gets a relaxation response (a feature hitherto dismissed as the placebo effect). These alone may be sufficient to switch the patient into healing (Pert, 1997) by boosting the autoimmune response. Hippocrates commented that some people will recover simply because of their satisfaction with the goodness of the doctor. Florence Nightingale famously described nursing as 'putting the patient in the best condition for nature to act' (Nightingale, 1869). In other words, something about the way we are with patients may be as significant, if not more so, than what we do. Being a healing presence, in healing relationship with another, may be the most powerful force toward healing. Indeed, when we enter such healing relationships, notions like patient and doctor, healer and healee, self and other, disappear. We may perceive, even for a brief moment, that mystical point when all once-firm barriers fall away and everything is present in the here and now, that sacred space where 'you' and 'me' simply slip into being part of all that is and the healing moment is known.

Healing emerges from this space. That healing may or may not include curing, the resolution of a particular disease. Indeed it is quite possible to die and yet be healed. Healing, with its roots in the Germanic word *haelan* meaning hale, whole or hearty, concerns our sense of wholeness, of being connected with the self and that which is beyond the self. An illness may be terminal, but we are healed because we have lost our fear of death, have resolved old hurts or see ourselves at last as more than the brief flash of our worldly existence. Healing can mean simply 'feeling good about myself for the first time in ages' as one chronically ill patient I have been working with recently has said. He went on to 'give up the drink' and get a job and renew many of his relationships. Technically speaking he is still a sick man and his physical illness is little changed. Yet he is different in the way he is now being in the world: more confident, more participative, more active, more whole.

THE HEALER–HEALEE TRAP

The last few points I have just made rarely fall within evaluation criteria for clinical effectiveness. The patient feels better, goes out and gets a job, enjoys his relationships more – yet these do not count. Technically he is still ill. His underlying physical status is much the same. I have a hunch that with continued work even this could change, but for the time being what has happened to this patient is without much of the criteria for measuring successful treatment. His 'results' don't match many measurable outcome scales currently used in the arena of randomised controlled trials or quality assurance tools. While it is generally recognised that evidence has its limitations (Feinstein & Horwitz, 1997) and that much of the process and outcome of healing is 'ineffable, mysterious and indefinable' (Abbot, 2000), this still leaves much of the current knowledge and research on healing beyond the scientific pale.

While it may be possible, as Abbott has argued, to research healing within the orthodox scientific paradigm, it may not only turn out to be impossible to explore in all but its limited manifestations; indeed it could also be counterproductive. Like the butterfly pinned down for examination, its exquisite beauty can now be made visible, but it has become a dead butterfly. Perhaps a vital aspect of healing is that, in order to be effective, it must be mysterious. Furthermore, is research into healing just playing to the agendas of others? Would discovery of the modus operandi of healing make more healing available to more people? Is it done to fit with the positivist assumptions about research, namely that if we do so we will be better able to cost it out, apply resources, improve training and accessibility, etc.? Perhaps other agendas are at work, such as the ego-driven need to be certain about everything. On the other hand, scientific research in the past has often led to more, not less, wonder at the creation. Certainly, seminal work of people like Jeanne Achterberg (see Chapter 5) would seem to make this possible.

Meanwhile, those who practise as healers, and call themselves such, risk limiting the arguably wondrous force they are working with. Healing is core to health care and part of every healthcare practitioner's work to some degree, whether consciously so or not. Yet, aggravated by wariness of examining or even talking about healing (or simply using 'healing' interchangeably and confusingly with 'curing') in orthodox circles, notions of healing seem to have become colonised almost entirely by the complementary therapies movement. Healing itself is emerging as a separate therapy in its own right. This may be seen as a worrying trend if healing is deemed something that certain (nominated) healers do, while others get on with some other part of the patient's health care. Thus arrive at the farcical situation of 'I go to my doctor for this, my aromatherapist for that, my healer for . . .' In other words, we end up with a mere extension of the reductionist medicine so prevalent now. If healing is core, not complementary, to health care, then why has it been lost or at least so much diminished from the mainstream? And can we get it back?

A more worrying trend is the claim put forward by some healers that *they* can relieve or heal injury and illness, often against the odds of medical prognosis (Charman, 2000). This is fuel to the fire for the sceptics, who dismiss the claims of the healers because no causal agent can be identified. Healers reinforce this division when they say that *they* are involved in a cause–effect relationship, between healer and healee, when *they* apply intention to heal and use the 'power of healing' as a therapeutic agent in its own right (Charman, 2000). Regardless of how this power is interpreted (light, love, energy, etc.), the tendency is for those who call themselves healers to see *themselves* as the channellers or guides or transmitters of this force in some way from, by or through *them* to another. I have used the italics here to emphasise the essential reductionist approach at work, not much different in fact from the much-maligned orthodox medical model – me doctor, you patient; separateness is not holism. In this model, only the 'therapy' has changed; the healer is just as separate from the healee as other labels of nurse or doctor or therapist *and* patient.

I get caught in this trap regularly and I expect many others working in healing ways experience the same thing. People come with their distress because they have heard someone is a 'healer'. When encountering someone suffering this is hardly the place and time to get into complex ontological debates about what is going on in healing. It is necessary to work with the person 'where they are' – their expectations and understanding, accepting given labels and roles (which may indeed be necessary to the patient's healing process). They can be appropriately explored in more depth later on, when deepening the patient's awareness of what is taking place may be part of their healing. From this may come an empowering realisation that they can be a significant determinant of their own health as active participants in the healing process, not merely passive recipients, and reach for themselves for a moment an understanding of the wonder that is healing.

The important point is that, while working with vernacular terminology, those who work with healing do not allow themselves to get caught up in the arrogant, ego-driven posture that they somehow heal another. Quite simply, they do not; nor do they have any evidence that they do. Something happens. It may be down to some subtle energy that we have yet to properly research and identify. It may be the result of some as yet hidden bodily self-righting mechanism or something special about human consciousness that we have yet to define. It may be God at work. We simply cannot be sure – except by the certainty that faith and experience can bring, but these have yet to be adequately tested in any randomised controlled trial. A healing response may emerge that we can witness, but its cause is essentially ephemeral. It is the stuff of involvement *with* the patient in the search for healing and the necessary entering of a place of (as yet) essential mystery. We simply do not yet have the tools or the evidence to exactly, incontrovertibly say what it is that takes place (though everyone working with healing probably has their own personal view) – to do otherwise leads to the scoffing of the sceptics and the fooling of ourselves.

What seems to be critical about healing work is the intention towards healing, and the coming together of one or more persons in search of healing (although work on non-local healing suggests that it is not even necessary for the persons to be in the same physical place together, as we have seen in Chapter 5). Thus by focusing our attention on healing, we enter a different world of healing, replete with potential. This is not a passive world of praying for the best or laying on of hands, standing back and expecting God to do the rest. Nor is it a world of the healer conducting the healing orchestra. It is a world of mutuality, of participation, where what seems to count is that we consciously join in the process, reuniting with that whole of which we are an equal part.

OFF WITH HIS HEAD!

I am blessed with the professional title of 'nurse', but paradoxically I learned long ago that I became a much better nurse when I stopped being a nurse. In other words, when I let go of my professional role and agendas (in my own head and heart, if not among the normal expectations and discourse with colleagues and patients). A patient with a back pain could see an orthopaedic surgeon and be told it's a disc problem; see a psychologist and be told it could be stress related; another therapist will say it's the product of pent-up emotions; someone else would see a blocked chakra; another a playing-out of karma; another a wound from a past life . . . and so on and so on. It's all down to whatever spectacles of a particular therapeutic model the practitioner is wearing. Illness is not just about suffering, but may have deeper purposes that the spectacles we use to view the patient obscure. Indeed, we have to be cautious that what we see may be simply a reflection of our own image in the glass of our viewer. We can simply never be sure what the healing entails for another. Beyond cures and our natural human desire to see another person well, we simply do not know the healing path of another; it is forever veiled to us, although sometimes the 'healer' may catch a glimpse when the veil is lifted.

A double-edged blade thus cuts right through the potential of healing. It cuts to the left by limiting the view of the practitioner to the enormous potential of healing when we see only one dimension of it through our narrow-range spectacles. It cuts to the right and severs our holistic connection to the other, simply because he or she becomes *other* when we set ourselves apart as a particular healer or health practitioner.

In healing, something happens. There are discernible outcomes, in terms of health and wellbeing, which happen to people as a result of experiencing healing. Our instincts are to search for the something. Is it some as yet undefined source of energy? The will of God? The impact of non-local consciousness? All of these and more? I have noticed a few common features among those who work in healing.

- A deep sense of humility by the healing worker who tends to shun the label 'healer'.
- A recognition that they can only describe a small part of what takes place and, even then, that words are inadequate.
- That they, along with the patient, are participating in something of which they are a part, yet is also much greater than them.
- That they are not in control of it. It works with them, perhaps because they are consciously participating, but whether or not it would be 'better' without them is an unknown.
- There is a sense of inevitability, of fate about the work. The one seeking healing has come together with that person at the time that is somehow right for them. They have 'chosen' at many levels, conscious and unconscious, to come together.
- They are not attached to outcomes. They recognise their natural human desire to want someone to be well, but see this as something to set within a wider context. They tend not to pray or ask for a disease to be cured, but wish for the healing and wholeness of the other, whatever form that might take.
- They rest in their work without the need for certainty or absolutes.
- They are fairly 'well-rounded' human beings, having worked on the healing of themselves, their ego attachments and so on, to enable them to be more relaxed and available with another without their own 'stuff' (such as the desire for power) getting in the way.
- They are very conscious of the quality of relationships in the healing process and its mutuality.

We can all play around with our healing techniques, models of assessment, diagnostic tools and panoply of pills and potions. They work, to a degree, but may leave us as actors on the comic–tragic stage of those we see as others. How much more powerful is this healing work when we relax a little and let go of our fixed roles, agendas and blinkered vision. We can do our usual work by all means, but need to remember to find that place in ourselves where we can sit back and let it happen, in wonder. The tools and models are there to help and inform us, not to be the healing bane, trapping us in the Minotaur's maze, from which there is no escape. No one is healer, no one is healee. We are all in this together. We pursue certainty, when perhaps it is also necessary to rest in mystery.

Chapter 18
Beyond 'being with'?

I am part of all that I have met;
Yet all experience is an arch wherethrough
Gleams that untravelled world, whose margin fades
For ever and for ever when I move

'Ulysses', Alfred, Lord Tennyson (in Gardner, 1989)

Harry's tale

I have a particular patient very much in mind as I write, and am mindful of so much professional literature that describes the effective healing carer as being someone with the capacity to 'be with', to be a healing 'presence', as I explored in Chapter 6. And the man (I shall call him Harry, a change of name for the sake of confidentiality) has given me a linchpin to explore a dimension of healing that has hovered around in my work for some years. This is personal, so I could be wide of the mark, but . . .

It was supposed to be clinical supervision session, a chance for a small group of staff on the ward to see Therapeutic Touch (TT) in action with a real patient after months of training, to check out and share their experiences, and to develop their practice. An explanation to Harry's wife about TT left her feeling comfortable about Harry's participation and able to consent. He couldn't do so himself, after Alzheimer's and strokes paralysing both sides of his body – his broken body could tell little of what he did or did not feel or know.

I felt uncomfortable even before I met him. A slight ill at ease that comes from wondering what will happen next. Would he be OK through this? (I had concerns even though there is no record of anyone being harmed by TT; the worst thing that can happen is nothing at all! (Sayre-Adams & Wright, 2001)), what kind of demonstration would this be? Of course in TT terms, like almost all the healing therapies (whatever name they use), where we talk of holism and being part of all that is, it could be argued that I was already sensing what was going on with Harry. At some unconscious level we were already meeting (had already met?). But then again I could have just been nervous myself, although I didn't feel so, when I checked myself out.

Whilst carrying on a normal conversation with the group in the room, as we waited for Harry's nurse to wheel him in to join us, I was quietly centring myself, something TT practitioners do to prepare and maintain themselves before and during the practice of TT. To the rest of the world you are carrying on as normal, but you are simultaneously 'bringing yourself home'. For me, it is just a gentle turning inwards, functioning as usual, walking, talking, doing: but I am also attentive to my breathing, becoming quiet and still within, bringing myself to a place of gentle alertness, watchfulness, witnessing: a meditative state, a concentrated yet relaxed attentiveness, centred, simply resting in the moment – present and watchful.

Harry was pushed into the room on his reclining chair. Expressionless and frail, his body contorted by tightened muscles, a law unto themselves since the brain long ago abandoned control. I had prepared the seating for the group so that he would not feel surrounded. They were bunched into one corner, out of his line of vision. I hoped he would come to forget that they were there if their presence had registered with him at all. I was told he was wary of people and would become wild and distressed if anybody touched, approached or moved him.

I made a point of immediately sitting down next to him, eye level to eye level, and spent quite a while just sitting like that before I moved my right hand slowly forward into his line of vision, then to his left wrist (the moveable hand), and stroked the back of his hand ever so gently. I said my name and something like, 'I don't know if you can hear me or not Harry, but I'm going to talk to you in a normal voice as if you can.' I briefly explained about TT: 'This isn't going to hurt, no need to be afraid. I'll just pass my hands close to your body. I'll only touch you very gently if at all. You may find it relaxing, most people do. But we can stop at any time if you're not happy with it or if I feel some how it's not what you want'. All this was said between Harry's occasional breathy quiet wail, an opening of the mouth like a crying baby, yet soundless.

I held eye contact with him whenever I could, remained seated by him, stroked the back of his hand and eventually slipped my hand between his fingers, feeling his grip, which was surprisingly strong and firm. I noticed that grip and eye contact were often simultaneous.

What was he trying to tell me? Or was this just the automatic grasp of the body – the mind and reason and personhood long gone. That's what I was always taught about Alzheimer's and strokes. The brain dies, so that means the person dies too. I never felt right with that message. If you buy into that scientific view, that the brain is the repository of consciousness, the mind, from which our unique being as a person emanates, then when the brain dies is there no person left either? In such a dis-spirited world, why bother taking care of the body? If the mind and therefore the reason and the person are gone, the rest is just vegetable. Why do anything with it at all? Oh, we hang on in there, telling ourselves that it's important to keep caring and keep comforting until 'nature (sans antibiotics) takes its course'. Respect them for what they were; they fought in the war, struggled to raise us, paid their taxes; they have their rights; they were once human like us. (Once human? What is it to be human?) We think we can work it like that, keep going on that basis. But we are sieves. We leak. No matter what solid container for the rationale of our actions and beliefs we seek to construct, it's full of holes. Somewhere along the line, if I don't really believe that there is something in there, in or around that body, that remains watching and knowing, then my container is just a leaky vessel. I am holed by deeper disbelief that it's not worth bothering because it's just a body and there really is nothing else there. Then, at some time, behind the mask of human kindness and compassion, we may catch a glimpse of our deeper dis-quiet as it leaks out.

I think of countless cases where carers have abused older people. I think of the hospital in Irsee near Munich where the nurses and doctors killed the eld-erly and disabled patients during the war (*lebensunwertes Leben*, 'life unworthy of life'). That is the logical trajectory of rational thought. When the brain goes, the person goes. They become non-persons. When they become non-persons, those who care for them are tested. Can you see the person behind that bro-ken body, empty mind? (Bring in the photos, the wedding snaps, the love tokens – Ah yes, he loved like me, had a job, had a life.) Maybe I can see the person then. Be reminded. That way I'll keep it going, keep nursing, offer respect, dignity . . . But when I lapse. When I can't see the person any more. When the veil of pretence slips away and that deeper sense of 'I don't really believe this is a person' peeks through. When I can't see them as me any longer, when they become a 'they', a 'them' – then it starts. And then you can do what you want with 'them'. A little ignoring here, a minor infringement there. The conversation over the body. The silent bath. The mug of tea – sugar? – no matter . . .

In the mists of disconnection begins the slow drip of inhumanity, comes the stream of letting them go, comes the river of seeing them off, comes the dark ocean of the mercy killing fields.

This is where it starts, elder abuse, if at some level, no matter how we strive against it, in our deepest selves we don't really believe that there is anything wor-thy left, not brain or body, but personhood, being. No matter what the body represents – a remembrance of things past. If we don't really believe that there is more, then there is only less – and it's just not worth going on any longer.

They are gone (or going) and that's it. What's left is a body, nothing else: just an empty container, a bin liner for consciousness now empty – and less valuable.

. . . but to return to Harry.

There was something about the look in his eye while working with him, some intensity, some inner knowing that took me aback a little. I continued with the TT assessment, keeping eye contact as much as possible, passing my hands slowly along the length of his body just a few centimetres above his skin and clothes. He responded warily, seeming afraid of actual touch. I remember saying quietly and repeatedly, 'It's all right, it's OK, I won't hurt.' Using my hands was barely necessary; my intuition was in overdrive already. I kept having to pull back and centre myself, the impressions were so strong. His body felt utterly unbalanced – a deep hollowness of the lower half, searing pain along the right side especially. I felt drawn into him, into his experience, and his eyes . . . I just kept 'hearing': this is what it's like for me. To be inside this body. I was close to tears and struggling to stay centred. The pain was awesome. I had never experienced TT like this before, so intimately, so powerfully, so rapidly.

I was almost overwhelmed by a sense of what it was like to be Harry. I was *being* Harry. This was beyond being with him, beyond empathy or compassion or 'presencing'. There was no he and I. This was a kind of union. That place of mystery that I've heard about in healing work, where all the boundaries fall away and there is no difference between wounded and healer. We were both in the same place – and there was no we, no both, just being in the same place. It came and went, this feeling. At one moment there was just an immersion in oneness, at the next a re-separation, when I was flooded with imagery and impressions of what it was like to be Harry, to be holding that body. This was the place of knowing. I was rocked by the pain and the intensity of the impressions. I looked at him at one point and said, 'Oh, Harry, how do you go on with this? What a tough one, what on earth are you doing inside that one . . . ?' Suffering. A state of continuous suffering.

I felt like I was reporting back. Like somehow I was being informed of that which he could not speak. And I looked at him and thought, 'You know'. At some level he was not suffering himself. HimSelf. He was just watching all this. Experiencing it. Knowing it. Being in it. Yet in some way apart from it – witness and participant in one.

So I reported back. This was what we talk about in TT by mutuality. It's not one way. In TT we may get as much from a patient as they get from us. I was learning fast. This is co-creation – using what I was learning to feedback to others, which was going to mean, I knew, a radical rethinking of his care and rolling to the back of my mind so much of what was happening. Profound work to reflect upon later.

I tried to tell people what it was like for Harry. Here was suffering (yet at some level he was not suffering) and what could we do about it. I could be completely wrong. This was TT in full flow but I had no 'scientific' evidence to back me. Part of me was rationally dismissing the experience as delusion, illusion, confusion. Oh, I could quote the theory of TT, talk about the energy fields, the holistic universe and quote quantum physics ad infinitum – but I could still just have been crazy. What I was experiencing could simply have been the product of wild imaginings.

And yet Harry seemed so calm, held my gaze, and I could not escape this deep sense of knowing and the urge to respond to it. When we know there is suffering, then we can make choices. We can walk away from it, ignore it, or we can act. Then in a sense we are gods. Then we can make choices. I attempted to explain to my colleagues in the room.

> *You have to imagine what it is like for him. Every cell of his body feels to me to be highly charged. His vision and hearing are supersensitive. A ceiling light is brighter than the desert sun. The drop of a spoon on the floor sounds like thunder to him. A touch, like the blow from a hammer. Imagine a small burn or scald to your skin, just enough to peel off the top layer and leave a raw, wet, pink exposed layer beneath. Each nerve ending screams at you in pain. That's what it is like for him – all over. Pain. It is not dull or slow, it is fast and sharp – coming and going in waves. And he slaps his head as he always has because it hurts. He slaps his head to tell you this. He slaps his head to make it hurt to diminish the sense of pain elsewhere. When he slaps his head, he is speaking to you. And Him, almost overwhelmed by the limitations and strugglings of his broken body and his lost mind. But Him. 'Him' is watching every moment of this. Knowing that it is perfectly in its place. At some level he knows and is not suffering. He is simply present with absolute loving compassion at what is happening to this body and mind of his. He is not waiting or wanting. Just watching with utter patience . . .*

I was struggling to capture in words even the smallest sense of what I was experiencing and to convey it to others. I felt like some foreign correspondent, trying to get across the intricacies of a complex war to the comfortable audience in front of the TV screens back home.

I continued the mechanics of TT. Like all other therapies, TT is just the route inward – the technique which happens to guide one into the healing space; but it's also not about the technique. It's beyond that. Even that has to be let go of. We learn our technique, but that too must be put aside as we slip away into the healing sacred space and trust what arises. I used my hands to pass over his body, holding his left hand from time to time, 'saw' smoothing, filling, easing, rounded, wholeness . . .

He seemed settled somehow. It was time to finish . . . how long had we gone on . . . a minute? . . . an hour? . . . There was no sense of time or place.

And we talked. About what we do now. Some of the group were deeply moved. He had never responded like this before. One said, 'I feel almost guilty that everything I've done has got it wrong', and another, 'His wife always just sits with him. She never does anything – perhaps she knows more than us'. What we were suggesting ran counter to everything you do for 'dementia' patients – providing silence and solitude and dim light and peace and quiet – instead of all the razzmatazz of constant stimulation. Everything about how he was touched, moved, held; all that was done to him was going to have to be re-thought. If this was true. If TT was right. If I'd got it right. Who knows? I 'felt' I did. What we were proposing 'felt' right. And we all know what he was like before. And here he sat now so calm and quiet in the hands of a stranger, where hitherto he could have seemed wild. Who knows? Harry does. We turned his care plan on its head after that. Some of the staff took some convincing, but the change in his behaviour when we included more solitude, stillness, pain relief, dimmed lights, careful touch and TT sessions was the proof of the pudding. The transformation into long periods of rest and serenity was a world away from his previous wild reactions.

AND THEN

So much of healthcare theory speaks of companionship, partnership, being with, presencing, and in earlier chapters I have explored some of these concepts in detail. Yet all of these are fundamentally dualist. 'Practitioner' and 'patient' remain essentially separate – for safety's sake, as Campbell (1984) suggests when he writes of companionship as journeying with the other and being intimate 'but within defined limits'. So much about caring roles is constructed to protect the carer. It is assumed that by getting close, so close as to be an open and aware presence with the other, we can determine what care is best needed. For most patients, this may be all that is needed – 'sort me out please and send me home'. But perhaps there is something beyond this, some way of being that serves not only the patient but the practitioner too, at some deeper level. Beyond I-you, however empathetic this relationship may be, lies another realm of relating, where you and I disappear – a coming-together into a oneness, into union.

I mentioned this idea at a conference recently and heard the deep sigh of disbelief from some colleagues. Union? Impossible – we are physically and mentally always separate. True, but what I seek to suggest here is another realm of possibility. Not a bodily union, but an altered state of consciousness, a 'place of mystery' where all is one.

It goes against everything I have been taught as a nurse: always being separate. Not getting involved was considered essential to good practice. But this is beyond emotional involvement or overgiving or overworking . . .

It can't be safe for everyone. For to enter union requires a degree of maturity, of fearlessness, of loss of ego that permit merger, knowing fearlessly that individuation will return. There is a purity to this kind of work, a capacity to let go of ego needs and desires, firm concepts and fixed ideas, and just trust. There is discipline too; it cannot be reached without the hard and consistent ego work down the years. Like any healing or meditative practice, when you are a practitioner there has to be a steady stripping away of thoughts, desires and ego attachments, until you can come to a place that allows you not to be you, to let go of self and enter Self with trust and wonder. It is a humbling process, too, and liberating. The greatest thing our ego/personhood fears is annihilation, but as the mystic path shows, the annihilation of the ego's power is a setting-free. For when we let go of that, we in a certain way die, but this death is a little death of the ties that bind us to a limited concept of who we are. I become nobody, and only nobody enters sacred space. While I remain a somebody, I am forever kept on the periphery to some degree. Nobody gets into heaven! Annihilated into the greater self, we are set free. There is no need any longer to worry about 'being me', for 'me' becomes the instrument of my being in the world, just the instrument. 'Me' is conceived differently – I can let go of superhood, the need to be in control, the need for the power of survival and status. Fear dies, and fearlessly we are now able to enter the healing space (and can only enter it thus). I become not the healer (an illusion) but companion with the other along the way into the healing space. Perhaps 'I' am only the guide, the way-shower, for maybe I have less fear than the needy one. I am the escort into the place where healing lies and fear is dispersed.

Or maybe it is not about being a guide, but being guided, called at some level by the other from a faraway place (that is here, now) – 'Here I am, come and see.'

And healing at its very root is the extinction of fear. Healing is not just about making bits of the body better. It is the extermination of fear – letting go of it and becoming aware of who I really am. When that happens, the bodily journey is accepted as it is. Maybe an illness may be cured, maybe not, but I can be healed in this because the fear dies, for I know who I really am. I have come home to my true self. Healing in this sense is a preparation for death, of letting die all that we think we are, to discover who we really are.

So many healers and techniques and cults are set up as ways, consciously or unconsciously, of avoiding this. They work from the premise of being a something or a somebody. Holding you on to what it is that you think you are. Whatever you think you are, you are not. Surrendering into nobody is anathema to this view.

We enter this healing space together and for a brief moment, if time here means anything at all, we are not 'we' but one. It doesn't have to be embellished or enhanced, what we witness here. Although sometimes, in the struggle of our senses to make sense of it or the pride of the ego that seeks attachments and importance, we create labels and clever responses. 'An angel guided me', 'Red Cloud, a great medicine man, is my guide', 'I channel God's power' – all illusions, grasped at by the ego mind, which seeks control and certainty and existence. The experience of the sacred space of healing is a humbling experience, a humility that arises from the wonder of what we witness, the height and breadth and depth of the knowing of the unknown. And yet it happens because we are here, because we present ourselves, stripped bare; we are clothed in a kind of glory. We participate, we co-create. As we glimpse beyond the veils, there is a moment of seeing, in oneness, that it happens because we are needed as part of that oneness. Our nobodyness makes us exist! That is the paradox.

Underhill's (1993) classic text on mysticism offers us a model, from a different perspective concerning union with the divine, it is true, but with principles that may be transferable here. She describes five distinct stages described by all mystics. The first is 'Awakening', a sense of being called or hearing the voice of God that may change our lives dramatically. The second stage is 'Purgation', the period in which the person realises that they are not good enough. How could they possibly be called to do this profound work of service? So they try to purge themselves of worldly connections, often through fasting and extreme acts such as giving away their material possessions. The third phase, 'Illumination', is when the person is utterly filled with passion for and a sense of God. The fourth phase, 'Surrender', typically goes on for a long time. It is a very profound period in which the person explores their inner, divine connection. This period of spiritual development often includes much suffering because, as the person strives for perfection, they can never be good enough. The fifth phase is 'Union', during which the mystic realises that they have reached a level of deep inner connectedness with the Divine Reality; the two become one, 'advaita'.

Many people report such mystical union and it is probably far more common than is generally believed (Maxwell & Tschudin, 1996). Through life experiences, prayer, a chosen technique, drugs, relationships, contemplation, sex . . . or a brief moment with all these, we can experience a sense of loss of self, and union with something that is beyond the self. We could conjecture what impact there would be if our educational programmes for healthcare practitioners could once again include spiritual practices, to bring more of us to that place in ourselves where we are fearless and connected to the greater realm of being.

Such a profound process in relation to the connection to the divine may seem somewhat far-fetched, at first hand, in relation to the day-to-day experience of most practitioners and patients in the realm of conventional medicine. But it does offer a framework for exploring what seems to be a hitherto unexplored dimension of the carer–patient relationship, to take both towards healing.

It is not necessary for all carers and patients. The ordinariness of caring relationships is all that is needed in most settings – but another possibility now emerges for connection that seems to have been little explored in mainstream health care. The purpose here may not be to unite with the divine through the (painful) process of the five stages outlined by Underhill, but the principles may be the same, albeit applied at a different level.

For example, by undertaking a course in, say, psychoneuroimmunology or TT or some other complementary therapy, a practitioner may 'awaken' to the possibility of understanding human beings in a different way from the dominant biopsychosocial models. A form of purgation takes place as we realise that our old models are not good enough and do not have all the answers, and further, as this impacts upon our egos, we let go of superhood and the need to be in control. As with all healing work, ego work is a parallel exercise. Only when we re-examine and let go of our previous concepts of self are we able to enter fearlessly and safely a deeper union. This is serious work. It cannot be bypassed. There are no short cuts to the emotional work. It requires attention, discipline and commitment. Later, we may be illuminated by the emerging possibilities of working and healing in different ways than we have previously understood, and liberated by the awareness that loss of self is not a loss, but a freedom from so many constraints and restrictions. Surrendering, we die to the limitations of what we once thought we were, burn away the fear of intimacy and connection, and learn to watch in wonder at the potential for things to be done when we give up the desire for the power to do things. Cleansed, we can enter into union; having surrendered our wishes, expectations, hopes and agendas, we can simply be with the other, letting our therapy of choice be the vehicle to transport us to a deeper connection with the other, so deep that other and I disappear. Separation is an illusion. Words like I-we-you-me-they fall away as meaningless as we enter a place of mystery, of contradiction and harmony, of unity and separation. I am in this place where I and you are one, and yet I still see my 'I' and it serves, to understand, to recognise, to watch, to witness.

When the moment passes there is a knowing. I felt only wonder and gratitude in the example described above, one of many in my personal experience. And like the mystical path, the challenge now arises – what do I do with this knowing? Do I rest in bliss? Give up on the world and all its now seemingly small limitations? Or is it a case of 'after the ecstasy, the laundry' (Kornfield, 2000). In some way this process is empowering, but it is not ego or personal empowering. It is a humility process, a day off for the ego, a chance to see the nature of real power coming from a place that at first hand might seem powerless. To enter this place of mystery is to lose hope ('for hope would be hope of the wrong thing' (Eliot, 1944)), to surrender into possibility without personal control or expectation.

This is sacred space, a boundless altered state of consciousness where all potential is contained, the void from which every creative possibility emerges, boundless once our own ego is laid to rest. Only who we think we are binds us. Lose the self and we find the Self. We enter it, we dance with it, we return to ordinary reality with new choices, new patterns, new visions, pregnant with the possibility of co-creation. Only with the humility of the stripped-away ego can we make right choices, and make right relationships for healing. We do and we do not do. This is the realm of the unity, the One, the diamond conscious-ness, the sky of mind. It is the womb of Isis, the vast and borderless chamber from which all flows.

Can we teach this to others? Yes, through all manner of programmes, not least the approach to TT. Awakening, purgation, surrender, illumination, union – these are the very stuff of deep learning, which transport us from the narrow confines of concepts of self and lead us by the terrifying path of loss of self, only to discover our true Self, our true being. We do not head towards union; it is not a journey in the movement sense. Instead it is a quietening, a stilling, a resting aside of who or what we once thought we were so that we can be utterly available to another. We paradoxically must work for it, yet also surren-der desire for it, for the desire becomes an obstruction along the way. It is the goalless goal. We must burn in our hearts to want it to happen, yet give up all desire to make it happen. Then it arrives, in a moment, when unexpected. We do not work to become somebody: we seek to become nobody – no-body and nothing, no-thing. Only then do we discover Somebody, Something. So, pro-grammes that do not just fill the practitioners' heads with new knowledge, but open their hearts to the potential that lies within, may transform the way we approach the path of healing for millions of people. The healing practitioner treads the same steps as the mystic, the same path to union – and at some level the place they arrive at is the same. For all healing emerges from this one, sacred space – the Absolute, the universal Consciousness, the primordial Source, God.

And when we return (not quite the same) to separate identities, as I did with Harry, then we can choose. Then things may be different. I can work to relieve suffering because it is not just determined by 'me'. Healing is a mutual process, a co-creative act. Maybe I have helped Harry – and you could dismiss it as weird stuff, fantasy, telepathy, call it what you will. But something has happened to both of us when we return from being in the place of union.

> This essentially relative to another, somewhat is virtually an other against it: since what is passed into is quite the same as what passes over, since both have one and the same attribute, viz. to be an other, it follows that something in its passage into other only joins with itself. To be thus self-related in the passage, and in the other, is genuine Infinity.
>
> Hegel, 1892

CHAPTER 19

POWER, PROFESSIONS AND PRACTICE — MUTUALITY AND GRACE IN HEALING WORK

Just as the person who comes to see me needs me for help,
I need him to express my ability to give help.

James Hillman, 1979

A GRAND ENTRANCE

She walked into the room like she owned it.

Her long, flowing grey hair was perfectly cut. Her immaculately co-ordinated attire fell about her tall and elegant frame. Her manner and bearing left no doubt that here was a woman sure of herself. People gave way to her, deferred to her, appeared diminished in her presence. Her students gathered about her, scurrying to fill her glass, checking her comforts, almost bowing when addressing her, seeming to vie for her attention. She cut an impressive presence.

Her words when she spoke were a revelation. She reeled out the lists of patients she had cured and held the audience enraptured by her tales of her healing powers, how she directed and worked the 'energy', how patients were transformed in her hands. The seduction of the audience was completed with the assurance that they too could become great healers in the certainty of the teaching she offered.

As the applause gathered momentum, I quietly left the room.

She could have been any New Age healer or for that matter a conventional physician. So much of the healing/curing dialogue is wrapped up in notions of powerful people able to use their skills, of whatever type, to do things to or upon or for others in a linear process from them to the other. In all the talk of holistic care she purported to offer, here was someone still trapped in outmoded notions of the nature of healing relationships. It was still one way, still from her to the other. As I suggested in Chapter 17, healing is not about personal power, in fact quite the reverse. Health practitioners, through their deepening awareness and spiritual practices, learn to let go of their agendas to be in charge, to fix things.

I work a great deal among what might loosely be called New Age healers, mainly complementary therapists, and I've noticed among not a few an over-weening attachment to their therapy and the certainty that they have got it right – the very thing that many such practitioners would accuse their ortho-dox colleagues of – and thus are caught up in the very webs of self-deceit for which they often condemn conventional medicine. However you dress it up, the language of the professional healer or carer, whatever the type, can so often be used 'to obscure the issue of power' (Hugman, 1991). Just because someone is a complementary therapy practitioner, there is no guarantee that they are any less addicted to their own self-importance than those in orthodox medicine.

There is a sort of denial at work here too. I am not so sure that the lady in question had the insight to see what she was getting out of her relationships with patients. But feeding off them she certainly was. Leaving aside the issue of deriving an income from her healing work – I have no problem with that – she was also gaining in other ways. Her ego was feasting on the power over others, on their acclaim, on their gratitude, on the self-importance it generated, the feelings of control it nourished.

I guess I may be unfair commenting. Who am I to judge? If it worked for her patients, it worked. If she got a high out of her activities, then so what? I just have a little niggle at the back of my mind, though, a tiny voice squeaking mouse-like in the shadowy recesses of my perceptions that at some level the healing processes in her work were being inhibited. It was all very authoritar-ian and top-down. Somehow the patients and her students were very much junior partners to her. Her seductive certainty was, at some level, keeping peo-ple in a certain place beneath her – disempowered and incomplete   although they may not even have known it. In healing work there should be a sense of liberation; here I felt only a sense of binding. Maybe it doesn't matter. If folks were genuinely getting better in her hands, who am I to quibble? Yet the dis-quiet remained.

WE'RE ALL IN THIS TOGETHER

Arthur Frank's (1991) sometimes chilling account of his relationship with health professionals, through a heart attack and cancer, remains with me, although I read it over a decade ago. He graphically illuminates the sense of disconnection and dis-ease that comes from the apparently benevolent, yet inherently malev-olent, process of the exercising of power by health carers. When carers connect with him in open, honest and humble ways, his perceptions of his illness are transformed. Hope emerges out of hopelessness, confidence out of fear, control out of collapse. What the most effective carers seemed to possess was a deep recognition that in their encounters with their clients, the healing traffic was not one way. The carer was getting something out of the process too. I have been struck by how many carers I have encountered who are able to acknowledge this mutuality. Time and time again, I have heard doctors and nurses and therapists of all kinds acknowledge that a spiritual connection in their work is contained in that phrase, 'But I'm getting as much out of this as you are,' when faced with the grateful patient.

Mutuality, the concept that a rapprochement or an equal exchange exists in healing relationships, underpins the work of all of the most effective 'healers' (see Chapter 17) I have ever encountered. My friend and teacher Ram Dass speaks of 'suffering as grace' (2000) – an opportunity to use illness to deepen our connection with our deepest selves. Another friend, Gretchen Stevens, who works locally in an innovative centre for complementary care, has commented to me that the invitation to help someone in their suffering is also a kind of blessing or grace for the practitioner. This encapsulates the opportunity not only to express our own need to help others (as illustrated in Hillman's quote, above) but also to fulfil a wide range of other possibilities for ourselves when we enter healing relationships.

Alastair Campbell, a theologian working in Edinburgh some years ago, developed interesting ideas about the nature of professional relationships. He saw professionals moving away from the old-fashioned authoritarian and patrician approach to patients (based more on their needs for power over others or delusions of altruism). Right relationships with patients emerged as partnerships, with recognition of the mutual benefits for both parties. He saw such relationships as a form of 'companionship' typified by a 'closeness which is not sexually stereotyped' and which 'implies movement and change', expressing 'mutuality', and requiring 'commitment, but within defined limits'. He writes:

> Companionship describes a closeness which is neither sexual union nor deep personal friendship. It is a bodily presence which accompanies the other for a while. The image of the journey springs to mind when we think of the companion. Companionship arises often from a chance meeting and it is terminated when the joint purpose which keeps companions together no longer obtains. The good companion is someone who shares freely, but does not impose, allowing the other to make their own journey.   Campbell, 1984

It is interesting that many patients who have written about their illness experience use the word 'journey' to describe it, and the 'spiritual journey' is common parlance. While we are on the journey it can indeed seem to be a distance, perhaps a long distance, in time and place as we move from one experience to another. Interestingly, Meister Eckhart, the great Christian mystic, understands why it can feel like a journey, but adds that we can reach a point where we realise that the journey was only half an inch long, 'but a mile deep'. (Eckhart, translated by Davies, 1994).

We often encounter companions on journeys – people who we may help along the way and who may help us. The notion of mutual assistance is developed further in the many reports from therapists of many kinds that they, as well as their patients and clients, derive some sense of wellbeing from their healing encounters. One survey of Therapeutic Touch (TT) practitioners (Lewis, 1999) found that, as a result of practising TT, there was an increased sense of wellbeing, strength and energy, calmness, stress relief, centredness, personal reflection and so on. Similar findings are reported by Green (1998), who comments on the 'benefits to be gained for both the person giving Therapeutic Touch and the person receiving it'. A study by Quinn and Strelkauskas (1993) indicated a measurable improvement in the practitioner's immune response. I suspect that similar phenomena could be demonstrated with a whole range of therapies – both complementary and conventional. Rogers' (1990) updated theory of integrality points to the possibility of human 'energy fields' interconnecting to influence the wellbeing of each other. Indeed in Rogers' context, 'each' and 'other' are redundant concepts in an holistic universe. Clearly there is a great opportunity for theory development and more substantive research to be undertaken in this field, to underpin scientifically what many report anecdotally.

HEARING YOU I HEAR MYSELF

Barbara Dossey (2001) adds further evidence to support this argument. She speaks of the impact of patients relating their stories to nurses and comments that.

> *We are our stories! Every time we connect to a story, we connect with another patient, who comes alive for us. Connecting with the stories of others uncovers or reveals aspects of our own stories we've forgotten or repressed. That's why the stories of patients can help healthcare workers on their own journey towards wholeness. That's also why being called to the work of service in healthcare is such a sacred path and a spiritual journey.*

This echoes the comments of Gretchen Stevens (above) and is further reinforced by Frank (1991) when he returns to this theme and writes of the unique illness experience of each unique patient: 'When the caregiver communicates to the ill person that she cares about that uniqueness, she makes the person's life meaningful. And as that person's life story becomes part of her own, the caregiver's life is made meaningful as well.'

There is a caveat to all this, however. It is important to make a distinction between mutuality and co-dependence. If Hugman (1991) is right that professional relationships are deeply imbued with attachments to power over others, then the possibilities for abuse are enormous – as the litany of murderous and destructive acts by doctors, nurses and other health professionals has shown. Sometimes the patient–carer milieu is perverted to meet the needs of the carer, beyond the mutual recognition of participation in the healing process or to express the desire to be of help to others. It can be the context, as we have seen in Chapter 1, which allows the carer to act out the more sinister needs emanating from their shadow side, the space where the need to be needed can lead to exhaustion and burnout in caring relationships where mutuality is lost in the slide into co-dependency.

These reservations aside, it seems that the connection between two or more human beings in healing relationships is replete with possibilities of health and wholeness, and not just for the one we label the patient or client. Sometimes we may glimpse this sacred connection if only for a moment. For some people, and I count myself blessed at this point in my life to be among them, the experience is a sustained one. I find myself frequently with patients, wondering what on earth I am doing or even if I am doing anything at all! Something is going on, but I struggle to define it – perhaps I shouldn't even try. Perhaps, as I suggested in Chapters 17 and 18, the miracle of healing is diminished if we try to pin it down. I'm just left with a deep sense of awe, wonder and appreciation at what is taking place. Amidst a general feeling of wellbeing, a sometimes gloomy world can seem a little brighter that day.

CHAPTER 20

IN A BALLROOM MIRROR – REFLECTIONS ON SACRED SPACE

In a fair orchard, full of trees and fruit
and vines and greenery, a Sufi sat with
eyes closed, his head upon his knees,
sunk deep in meditation, mystical.
'Why,' asked another, 'dost thou not behold
these signs of God the Merciful displayed
around thee, which He bids us contemplate?'
'The signs,' he answered, 'I behold within;
without is naught but symbols of the Signs.'

Jalalu'uddin Rumi (cited in Friedlander, 2003)

A SACRED VALLEY

White-painted stone buildings are two a penny in Cumbria, the Lake District National Park, which is my home. You could pass each by and note its own unique qualities, yet after a while, they take on a kind of serial prettiness as each merges into one overall impression of a particular style. The Quaker meeting house in the village where I live is one such building, like thousands of others in this part of the world. A stranger, unaware of its content or purpose, would pass it by unremarked and unremarkable, like so many others hereabouts. But picture a band of tourists in their woollies and waterproofs, decked out for winter in the unseasonably warm spring sunshine and entering the musty silence of the meeting house. A silence hangs in the air among the dark oak benches and limewashed walls, the roar of a passing car or ecstatic songbird both equally hushed and distanced by the quiet of this place, a quiet that seems to spread way beyond this room, these old seats, these damp stones. It is as if some presence here holds a deep stillness that muffles anything that would encroach upon it. The violation of the outside world is held at bay here.

As we arrive, so we leave, returning to bright sunshine and the first thrust of daffodils under the sycamores and the noisy chatter of a tour recommenced. And then I pointed to the peak before us, the whaleback purple-grey hump of Carrock Fell rising right outside the door. On the sides of this fell are remnants of Neolithic tombs, and heaps of rocks around its crest testify to a place of ritual and ceremony, long deserted by the first peoples of these islands. As the ice receded and trees began to cover the land once more, people followed: hunter-gatherers first, who left few signs; then, perhaps six or seven millennia ago, settled farming communities, who marked the land with their tombs, henges and standing stones. Letting your gaze wander from fell to meeting house, the eyes pass over six thousand years of human history, six thousand years where in one place but in different forms people have gathered in worship, searching out the sacred in their own time and in their own way. To be in a place of such continuity is a humbling experience.

SACRED SPACE IN SOLID FORM

Since people first began to be conscious of themselves, and perhaps of that which is beyond the self, places have been marked to demonstrate their special significance. Two distinct views seem to have emerged. First is the very idea of a 'special' place, separated perhaps by natural or constructed barriers, which was set apart and reserved for or dedicated to the gods and to worship. The Greeks had their *temenos*, which could be a sacred grove or temple, and religious traditions of all kinds emulated this idea of something set apart and reserved for spiritual attention. In fact the word *temenos* is derived from the Greek *temnein* – to cut off or separate. Thus temples, shrines, sacred precincts, churches, pagodas and meeting houses of all kinds have been developed down the years, and it is interesting that often integral to or close by these sites were places for the care of the sick. For the *temenos* was a sacred or holy place and the word 'holy' is closely related to the word 'whole', from the Greek *holos*. Hale, whole, hearty, healthy can all trace their linguistic ancestry to similar sources. 'Whole' refers to something that is entire, complete, in an undiminished state (Oxford English Dictionary, 1999). 'Holy' stretches out that concept to the only thing that is complete and entire unto itself, to which nothing can be added or from which nothing can be subtracted, or that which is seen as belonging to it – the 'it' being God. God and that which is of God is considered (w)holy. The Latin root *sacer*, which also means holy, gives us sacred, sanctum and sanctuary – that which is of God. Some places were considered so holy, so sacred, that there were temples within temples. Thus the Greeks had the *naos*, the Jewish temple the 'holy of holies' and the Christians the 'inner sanctum'.

Please forgive this short diversion into dictionary definitions, but it is important to see in the linguistic roots some common threads – that for millennia people have ascribed holiness to certain places, where they could get nearer to God or Ultimate Reality, however they perceived it. These places were often associated with places of healing, healing and wholing it may be recalled being derived from the same linguistic source. The sick would be brought to the holy place in the effort to make them more whole, for sickness was seen as loss of wholeness (holiness) at some level and only by intervention from divine forces, perhaps by bringing the sick into close proximity with the holy place, could healing be achieved. Houses of healing, of hospitality, from which the modern hospital is derived, were always associated with holy work. Indeed only relatively recently in the secular Western healthcare culture have hospitals been segregated from holy work. At best, the hospital may nowadays have a chapel set aside for worship or special ceremony. Religious and spiritual support have been relegated to the role of the itinerant chaplain; the rest of the setting has been stripped of any religious association. In part, this is done in an effort to reduce the risks of offence in a multi-faith culture or to emphasise the rational and secular nature of modern scientific health care. However, in addressing these sensitivities, perhaps the baby has been thrown out with the bathwater and a whole tranche of the human experience has been denied – the spirituality of health and healing.

There is a movement afoot to recover this ground, as I have suggested in earlier chapters – such as the creation of sacred spaces within hospitals, and the growing attempts to integrate spirituality in health care. Meanwhile, in our efforts to make our healthcare systems free of religious dogma and judgementalism, we have also rid them of a core element of the healing process. Most healthcare settings are dedicated to the worship of rational, scientific medicine, but in so doing we have left God out of it. Or perhaps, more accurately, we have created new gods – cost-effectiveness, waiting lists, evidence-based practice, to name but a few. The very essence of healing is about restoring a sense of wholeness. To keep God out of it, however 'God' is manifested or interpreted for individuals and groups, is to deny part of the human experience, and that is contrary to wholeness. In the broadest sense of the term, much of our healthcare system has become Godless, and yet religiosity and spirituality are integral to our wellbeing, as we have seen in Chapters 1. Inviting God, the Absolute, back, without trawling in the shadow side of religion at the same time, is a major task that lies ahead of us if our healthcare systems are to be truly holistic.

SACRED SPACE IS EVERYWHERE

I have suggested that one view of the sacred place is that of a specially designated setting being holy, with some places being more holy than others. There seem to be some advantages to this, not least because our commitment to prepare for, visit and worship at them forms part of the spiritual experience. Even a weekly visit to church can be a sort of pilgrimage; as we prepare ourselves and make the effort of the journey, we contribute to a gradual shift of consciousness, letting go of the distractions and attachments to the ordinary and everyday, to focus ever more deeply on contemplation of the divine and the deeper reality beyond mundane existence. Thus, whether a place is deemed holy or sacred or not is bound up with the consciousness with which we approach it. We have one of two choices: we can visit as tourist or pilgrim.

The tourist comes to examine, explore, admire or critique. The pilgrim comes in search of connection and transformation. The tourist is distracted from the spiritual experience because they have come to look, to stand and stare, yet essentially approach the object of desire from a place of separateness, of objectivity, standing forever apart from it. The focus of the tourist is of temporary distraction, to move on to the next attraction when interest has been fulfilled (or boredom takes over). The pilgrim comes with reverence, seeking merger and involvement with the holy place, to be made more whole through contact with it and to leave taking some part of that holiness back into ordinary life.

Two recent examples show us the pitfalls of the tourist approach – F Scott Peck's (1996) *In Search of Stones* and Mick Brown's (1998) *The Spiritual Tourist*. The former travels to famous sacred sites in search of a 'turn on' but is distracted if the appearance of the place disappoints. The latter moves from guru to guru to find one who 'has the answers'. Both come away dissatisfied, not realising the source of that dissatisfaction and blaming it on some inadequacy of the place or the person. They both miss the point – that the sacred is not to be examined: it is to be experienced. It cannot be experienced by remaining an objective observer or trying to pin the sacred down into some limited definition arising from their own ego agendas. An experience of the holy, by definition, is about a sense of communion, of coming together, of integration, of participation, of making the pieces of our lives into one.

Some places can move us because of the grandeur of their architecture or the beauty of the location or the richness of their history, where generations have worshipped. But this is only part of the process. If we seek to remain outside observers, as the tourist does, then the holy will elude us, for only the pilgrim is willing to surrender so that they may actually experience it. And pilgrims and tourists do not mix easily. The conscious approach of each seems to fundamentally clash. Quiet prayer can be difficult as the masses mill through St Paul's Cathedral in London. The ancient, revered sites of Glastonbury Tor in England or Uluru (Ayer's Rock) in Australia seem somehow desecrated (made un-holy) when people stream over them and drop their garbage or let their kids treat them as football grounds. At Uluru the Aboriginal people hold a vigil and ask tourists, peacefully, not to climb this antipodean *temenos*. We backed off in deference to their wishes, but hundreds had fun and games on the climb, took pictures, had picnics and climbed down again and wondered what all the fuss was about. A beautiful sunset? – yes; a spectacular view? – yes; but a holy place? – no, let's get back on the bus and head for the next one. Meanwhile the Aborigines stood there in quiet disappointment.

At Stonehenge, that iconic British sacred space, huge numbers of people come to stand and gaze. Those who wish to revere and worship there must now book (limited) private access time. The Devil's Tower in Wyoming, a site sacred to Native American peoples, is approached by vast car parks and a tourist information centre. There is no sacred space information centre. When the tourists had gone, I had the place to myself and watched a magnificent sunset bring to life those stunning basalt columns, immortalised in Spielberg's *Close Encounters of the Third Kind*. I was transfixed and transformed by the vision. Months later, as I lay on the lawn and gazed in awe at the mediaeval ramparts of Norwich Cathedral, I was struck by the soaring stone of the cathedral tower – and saw them momentarily as both the same. The one, the Devil's Tower, a vast block thrust skywards by nature, the other carved by my ancestors in these islands – yet both having a similar symmetry of form and purpose. At Grace Cathedral in San Francisco, the replica Chartres labyrinth sits by the cathedral doors. You can walk this amidst the roar of a busy city – and it seems not to be a distraction – and fully engage with the mystery of inner shift that the labyrinth can cultivate. Or you can wander, like the portly couple I observed, around its walkway and admire its design and complex structure. Pilgrim or tourist?

THE PLACE, THE PRESENCE OR THE PEOPLE?

Not long ago I had a conversation with a regular visitor to Glastonbury. She felt that the 'energy' had moved away from its sacred sites because too many people were now irreverently visiting. An Aborigine I met at Uluru felt that the tourists were 'desecrating' that which was holy to the native peoples, and soon it would 'lose its power and become a rock like any other'. The crowds milling round our great cathedrals can look not dissimilar to the crowds milling round those new holy sites, the shopping malls of our towns and cities. I have met football fans who think of their team's home pitch as holy ground. Perhaps they are all right, or all wrong, but in the dumbing-down of our understanding of what holiness and the sacred are, something is lost. Maybe some places are special, more holy, because of their design, for example through sacred architecture principles. Or maybe some places by their naturally occurring shape or location inspire the same feeling. Does the Quaker meeting house at Mosedale convey a sense of the sacred because of its ancient walls or simple oak benches, or its silence? Does my kitchen feel as sacred to me or any visitor as the crypt at St Paul's Cathedral or the desolate landscape of Death Valley?

Perhaps some places are indeed special because of their inherent qualities. Maybe some places are more holy than others because of something we feel there, rooted in our perception of their history or because of some geomagnetic forces that influence our brainwaves, or perhaps even a special accretion of divine grace. Perhaps some places become holy because generations have worshipped and prayed there. If prayer, as the research often suggests, can influence a person's well-being, why should a history of prayer in one place not make that place seem more powerfully holy than others? Perhaps it is one or the other, or both or neither. There is the story of the monk who became enlightened by watching his own turd disappear down the toilet. Or there is Guru Nanak, the founder of the Sikh faith, who while on a visit to Mecca, was challenged as he sat in the street with his feet pointing towards the Ka'aba, the holy of holies to Islam. He was told that it was an insult to God to point the soles of his feet that way. 'Tell me where God is not,' he famously replied, 'and I will point my feet there.'

SACRED SPACE IS ALL

One of the impacts of defining some places as sacred is that by inference we define others as less so. Thus we create a dualistic universe – the holy and the not holy. Rules and regulations emerge to help us differentiate between the two. For example, Olsen (1999) discusses the concept of holiness in the Bible, which 'in Leviticus has two dimensions. The first dimension is holiness as separation. The sacred is separate from the ordinary or common. The holiness of God as a divine being is separate and distinct from humanity.' The second dimension of holiness is that of 'a goal' to which we should strive. The holiness of God becomes a model to be imitated – 'You shall be holy for I the Lord your God am holy'. (Leviticus 19: 2). Holiness in Leviticus becomes something we can aspire to if we follow certain prescribed actions. It is therefore less concerned with being an abstract concept and more about the way we organise our lives and conduct ourselves. This view is commonly found in all the great faiths, but also within these faiths and among others a different perspective is also offered. Jesus, for example, emphasised the kingdom of God as being 'within' – more about who we are, the nature of our consciousness and intentions, rather than in observable rites and rituals. In the Upanishads, that great Hindu spiritual text, 'everything, absolutely everything, is pervaded by the divine' (Easwaran, 1988). Pym (1999), writing of the Quaker tradition, notes that:

> Most religious systems have a concept of 'sacred space'. Churches, temples and other buildings dedicated to worship are blessed or consecrated. For Quakers, sacred space is created by the intention to meet together to experience the presence of God. It comes from within the worshippers.

Thus we see a shift in the concept of the sacred space – it is not just about special places, or 'everywhere', but also 'within' people. Whether something is sacred or not seems to depend largely upon the consciousness with which we approach it. Those things we designated as sacred, from our places of worship to the crystals in a New Age therapy room, may serve to shift our consciousness towards the sacred as we contemplate or make use of them. A sacred space is something that moves our consciousness, our attention and our intention towards God, and that could be anything, anywhere. It's just that some places or things – by their aesthetic qualities, by their ritual significance, by their history – are more likely to help than others. Whether we gaze upon a stone circle, or a beautiful sunset, or a scene of destruction, or the trash in the street we may be moved to the holy not by the thing in itself but by the way we think about it. Places and things can awaken the sacred in us, but to be awakened it must already be there! Do they do so by the special 'powers' they hold or do they do so because something in ourselves is lying ready to be birthed? Perhaps both. Perhaps what we attribute to the power of place is really only a projection of what is within us, but we deny it because it's so unbelievable that we can be that powerful ourselves. Thus we speak of the healing power of nature or a shrine, when its only real healing power is what we invest in it to trigger our inherent capacity for holiness, for God.

Exoterically the holy of holies may be the inner sanctum of the temple. Esoterically, the holy of holies lies within each of us, what George Fox described as 'that of God in everyone' (cited in Pym, 1999). Thus the issue is less about special places being sacred, more about the way 'we live sacredly, work sacredly and understand sacredly' (Palmer & Palmer, 1997).

Douglas-Klotz (1999) develops this idea further, suggesting that sacred space is not so much created as recognised. The space we create to acknowledge the sacred lies within ourselves when we set aside other concerns, as in prayer or meditation, for example, which opens us to an awareness of the Divine, the Absolute or the Highest Self. It is a place of an altered state of consciousness in which the holy is perceived and from which holy actions and intentions flow. He notes, 'In the end, it doesn't so much matter where we start as *that* we start. Holiness is about wholeness. When we allow something to be sacred for us, to remind us of the ultimate mystery, that something can lead us to every-thing.' Sacred space is therefore a conscious remembrance.

This remembrance helps us to keep our egos out of the way when we work in health and healing. It takes our role away from being the controller of the patient's fate and into being the midwife of their healing. Guenther (2002) writes of the 'ministry of presence', where our role is to be like a midwife, being a loving presence and available to the other , for the one who comes to us for healing is pregnant with their own capacity for healing. We do not heal them as much as help them give birth to their own healing. The sacred, the holy, is the space within and between us where concepts like within and between lose their meaning. There is just this moment, this boundless yet intimate space where every-thing is made whole.

THE BALLROOM MIRROR

I got laughed at, and sometimes punished, as a teenager for my daydreaming. I wasn't daydreaming but doing what I later realised was falling into an inner reverie, in communion with something that was beyond me yet intimately present. These experiences happened anywhere and everywhere: on a bus, in a church, in a classroom. I stopped trying to tell people about them because they only giggled or looked confused or got angry, or told me I was crazy. Only years down the line was I able to put words to it, this mystical, this numinous, this transcendent state. They told me then that to get to God you had to go to church. That was the only way.

But once, in the working men's club before the crowds arrived, I sat and watched the disco lights shimmer in the revolving mirror above the dance floor. I stood beneath it and saw bits of me and the room and the view outside gather and fracture in the mirror as it slowly turned. Each bit was a part of the whole, each bit had part of the picture, meaningless in their individual facets, but meaningful in their entirety. And it was the same feeling as in the bus or the church or the classroom. The tacky, beautiful, glittering mirror suffused into one radiant whole.

Sacred space is like that, irreducible in its nature. We may shift our perspective on it, see angles and aspects here and there, dance with parts of it. But to see it all, we must stand back and see its inherent wholeness. And even then its full nature and purpose may elude us; but mystery is part of the whole too.

CHAPTER 21

THE GIFT OF THE DEAD

A woman I knew just drowned herself
The well was deep and muddy
She was just shaking off futility
Or punishing somebody
My friends were calling up yesterday
All emotions and abstractions
It seems we all live so close that line
And so far from satisfaction.

Mitchell, 1976

THE RAW EDGE OF GRIEF

The notion that suffering is meaningful and purposeful can seem ludicrous when we are caught up in it ourselves, and one of the greatest of sufferings is bereavement. A personal experience of this recently brought these ideas into sharp focus.

We gathered round as friends and family do. The house, normally a quiet place, a home in which they were long accustomed to being alone together, was now full of people. Doorbells rang as neighbours called round or flowers arrived. Kettles boiled. Cups were filled, emptied, washed and filled again. This was a time of passing, when someone inconsolable in her grief, drowning in pain and confusion, was surrounded by people, some sitting in silence, others creating distraction with the making of sandwiches, or busying themselves with the answering of the door or the making of telephone calls. Death was in the air. Speaking and silence – painful not-knowing-what-to-say silences were punctured with conversations hung on uncertainty of the right words, and relieved by opportunities to give practical advice, something to say to fill the space, what to do and what not to do. People moved in and out of rooms, the flushing of toilets upstairs mirroring the flushing of words, memories and reminiscences, downstairs. The ebb and flow of 'emotions and abstractions'. The comings and goings, the making of plans and organising of things – funerals, money matters, security, who will stay, who will go – the pattern of normal life broken inside, while outside, through the net curtains and the wet hedgerows, it continued, cars passing, women with shopping bags with children in tow, a queue for the bus, an aircraft overhead trailing vapour lost to the wind. Ordinary life going on, bypassing the isolated cauldron of the home, now an island of un-normality, the death dance around grief to the tune of tears and the rhythm of despair; a capsule of life now set outside of life.

In the inconsolable grieving timelessness at the point of death, the left-behind living wail in disbelief, rail at the unfairness of loss, struggle to rethink a future where all plans, all certainties, all assumptions have been struck down. People, especially the most-loved of the dead, are rocked by confusion and the assault of uncertainty. Liferafts drift by for us to cling to – insurance to sort out, a phone call to be made, a funeral to plan, someone we had forgotten to notify to be tracked down. Practical things fill the timelessness with time, 'doing' fills the void of feeling. And in the midst of it all – she who is greatest bereaved, after a lifetime of devotion to one man, is now cast down and directionless in an ocean of loss and sorrow, feeling the utter aloneness that comes when the presence of love and companionship are irretrievably amputated by death. She falls, as the bereaved do, into the shocking, ice-cold realm of disconnection, into the hyper-pressure of the bottomless black pit where all light and life are extinguished, the abyss where nothing penetrates and everything is crushed down and collapsed into the tiniest, trapped, deadweight of unfathomable, soul-breaking, relentless pain.

A death in the family knocks us into another reality; ordinary life, with its passions and priorities, is put on hold. Although we may distract ourselves with things to do, with things to say, they are but momentary needlehooks of time grasped in a void where time and space can suddenly mean very little. No words of consolation – no matter how well meant or expressed – can fill this emptiness. Nothing done can take away the underlying pointlessness of action. This is a time of grieving when all words and doings fall away. Despite our best efforts to say and do the right thing (as much to make ourselves better as anything), feel useful or relieve the pain, this is a time when all that we can really do, beyond attention to practicalities, is simply be with the bereaved who sit on their mourning bench alone. The best we can do is come alongside and just be with them (Wolterstorff, 1987). The usefulness of doing pales into insignificance at this time, relative to the power of being, the capacity to be fully present with the grieving in their grief.

The vicar called in, alerted by the funeral director that there was a death in the community. He meant well, but his words to a numbed woman long since alienated from religion went through the air like the dust particles dancing in the ray of sunlight passing through the curtains. Some nodded in agreement to his words; others stared silently and vacantly at the wallpaper, seeming to find something there of riveting and profound meaning that had never caught their attention before. I left the room to take deep breaths from the cold spring air.

LIVING WHILE DYING

There was not a little anger directed at the vicar. The usual mutterings in quiet corners of the house – being English, no one was up-front enough to say it aloud, to the man's face. But there was anger there nonetheless – 'If there's a God, then why did he have to die like that?' and 'There's no justice, she didn't deserve to lose him like this.' Fortunately the good vicar, doing his best, had the good sense not to try and get into theological debates. He seemed to realise, at the last, that comfort is a dish often best served in silent presence – just hearing the pain without advice or attempts at rationalisation.

Western culture often stands accused of not preparing us for death (Kubler-Ross, 1969), seeing it as a time of loss or defeat, particularly among those influenced by some more limited views of Judeo-Christian and Islamic theology, which envision only one lifetime in this reality and consignment to heaven or hell thereafter. Such views are not universally shared in these faiths, but allied to Western materialism, they provide a fatalistic, toxic mix of short termism and fear. Other faiths such as Buddhism and Hinduism have different perspectives on the nature of this reality, a perspective largely shared by the mystical traditions of Judaism, Christianity and Islam (Teasdale, 2001). The Upanishads, that great Hindu mystical treatise, remind us that 'our native state is a realm where death cannot reach' (Easwaran, 1988). Buddhism pursues this thread, teaching that death is part of life in the cycle of death and rebirth but, in the end, having attained Nirvana, death is not loss but freedom: '. . . in the final fourth stage Nirvana is attained,' when 'the burden of the ego, the burden of life, has fallen for ever, and man is free' (Mascaro, 1973). The Dhammapadda, the core guidance on Buddhism, teaches that at this stage of enlightenment 'The traveller has reached the end of the journey! In the freedom of the Infinite he is free from all sorrows, the fetters that bound him are thrown away, and the burning fever of life is no more' (Mascaro, 1973).

However, the fever of life while it holds us in its grip is mightily difficult to let go of and, indeed, Eastern teachings have often been corrupted in the West to suggest that somehow, in attaining the enlightened, blissful, non-attached state, we can be free of all human connection and suffering. On the contrary, the reverse may be true – while becoming free we may also participate ever more deeply in (the pain and joy of) the human experience. Spiritual teachings are not designed as comforters, spiritual condoms to protect us from the suffering of life and death, but to connect us more deeply to it with ever greater compassion and awareness. The suffering is not necessarily lessened, but our awareness of it, and the possibility of a grander reality, change our reaction to it. There is a story of some Zen students walking through a village one day when they come across their great master bent in grief and sorrow over the body of his dead son, weeping inconsolably. The students approach him, puzzled and confused after all he has taught them. 'Master, master,' they exclaim, 'why do you weep? Did you not teach us that life and death are illusions, and there is not need for us to be sorrowful?' 'Yes,' replies the master, 'but the death of a child is the most terrible and sorrowful illusion of all.'

The suffering of death is unavoidable, indeed necessary, to help us shift from one perspective or reality to the 'real' reality. In this sense death is not so much dying from life as dying into it. 'It is a death to the false self, the egocentric life. It is the abandoning of the falseness to which our society habituates us' (Teasdale, 2001). The experience of all forms of suffering and death in life become the fire which burns off the ego attachments, our illusory grasping at one understanding of reality, freeing us for Nirvana, divine union, reintegration with Source. The Arabic term for this is *fana* – annihilation, non-existence, the stage we must pass through, as Rumi describes, in order to reach subsistence, union with the divine.

> *No one will find his way to the Court of Magnificence (Paradise) until he is annihilated . . . You are your own shadow – become annihilated in the rays of the sun (God)! How long will you look at your shadow? Look also at His Light . . . Come into the garden of annihilation and behold: paradise after paradise within the spirit of your own subsistence.*   Rumi, cited in Chittick, 1983

Spiritual practice in all traditions has at least one common thread: the preparation 'for our eventual encounter with death and what follows, whether this is conceived and experienced as heaven or some form of paradise, transcendence of the human condition subject to samsara or rebirth, or some other ultimate state of realisation' (Teasdale, 2001). The mettle of our faith and practice, of whatever tradition, is tested when we encounter in ourselves or others that point of crossover into the ultimate mystery. Religiosity contains the groundwork for that encounter.

READINESS IN THE DEATH FILE

I found a recent exercise in preparation for the ultimate encounter quite interesting. It was no grand scheme – just what I at first thought to be a simple activity – but it pressed many buttons for myself and others! I am now 55 after all, and I am likely to have fewer years ahead of me than behind me. The departure of children into weddings and the arrival of grandfatherhood in recent years have somehow focused my mind on what my loved ones would make of the deep chaos of my study. So, inspired by one author (Reoch, 2001), I set about creating my very own 'death file'. I've no plans to go just yet, but . . .

It sits in the bottom drawer of my desk and I am slowly making those who need to know aware of its content and location, though reactions are curious – from 'Oh, how sensible' to 'Oh, what's wrong with you?' I have promised myself to add to it and to keep it up to date. It's an interesting spiritual practice along the lines of the Buddha's teachings – about death coming without warning and making life in part a preparation for it. It has provided me with some degree of letting go and perhaps is an act of kindness for those who will have to clean up after me. Indeed, it could be argued, if we cannot face up to our own death, how on earth can we give fully to those who are actually dying or bereaved?

I have lost count of the number of grieving people I have nursed, whose lives at the time of (often) great trauma are burdened by the added difficulty of sorting out someone's finances and final wishes. With nothing in writing or no previously expressed views, sorting out what to do best can be immensely difficult, especially if death has been sudden and unexpected.

I began with the obvious; my will and my living will are held in a bright blue file marked 'My death'. Try that for starters: just try writing the words 'My death' on a file and envisioning what you would want to put in it, and see what happens! It means that you can't wait for illness; you have to start thinking about it now. Creating a death file forces you to take stock, both of your possessions and your aspirations, and to take the trouble to keep it up to date from time to time. It's easy to update your address file – but your death file too?

I looked at the paper trail of my life and asked what everyone needed to know to sort out my effects and wishes. So it's filled with birth certificates, insurance and credit card details, bank numbers and all the usual things that are often difficult to track down except by the owner. I've added contact lists and business matters that might need sorting, and the whereabouts of invoices and contracts. I've put notes in to my kids and other loved ones, instructions about what to destroy, give away or keep, and lists of myriad minor facts about everything from where to find my diary to where I store the hen food and how much to give them! (Perhaps my next area for spiritual practice should be on control-freakery!)

Collating the facts to smooth the path (if only slightly) after death for my loved ones is, of course, only half the exercise. As Reoch again reminds us, citing the Mahaparinirvana Sutra:

> *Of all footsteps, that of the elephant is supreme.*
> *Of all meditations, that on death is supreme.*

He goes on to point out that 'to work on our death file we need determination and patience' for 'fascinating questions start to present themselves. If we are prepared to be generous after our death, why not now? What would we regret not having done if we were to die suddenly? Do our life's priorities need to change?' (Reoch, 2001).

Preparing my own death file has emerged as a curious experience I had not previously considered. It is practical in outcome yet laden with spiritual dimensions. Try it. I recommend it. Those of us who work with death and dying have an investment in turning over the compost heap of our own issues around our own death — the more we sit at ease with our own, the better we are able to sit with others when they have need of us on their mourning bench. The helper's capacity to give care at the time of death may be directly proportional to the extent with which they are at ease with death themselves.

DEATH — THE GIFT

Readying ourselves for our own death may be a lifetime's process; not a subject of morbid fascination, but a conscious exercise with both practical and spiritual implications. Doing so in order to make death and bereavement less painful for ourselves and others seems one level of approach, doing so in order to deepen our awareness and annihilate the illusions of the self, or of mortality, quite another.

To those of an atheistic view, especially if that view precludes any possibility of another reality (the 'real reality' as the Upanishads describe), then the opportunities seem polarised between two extremes. If 'this is all there is', then we can either make a decision to be the best person we can be during the brief flash of our existence, or we can opt for a hedonistic line and exploit the world (regardless of the consequences) to gain maximum pleasure before our time is over — it is down to us. Such a (to some) depressing scenario is still a minority view in a world where many surveys, as was discussed in Chapter 1, indicate that the great majority of the world's population have some sort of 'there is more than this' values influencing their lives. Some scientists have suggested that the perspective of an afterlife or other reality may have been genetically determined, a defence in the face of worldly suffering, as explored in Chapter 00. The mystics, anyone who has had a numinous experience, those who have arrived at Truth through rational deduction or those who simply rest on faith would disagree — to them, God, the Source of All, the Oneness, is very real, as is the reality of an afterlife or a dimension of reality, beyond ordinary reality, where rests the immortal, the eternal.

The disciples asked Jesus about death, and like all great spiritual teachers he did not provide a straight answer. Rather, he stretched them by offering a tantalising glimpse of a different possibility, which they would have to work at to understand. In so doing, he completely subverted their existing notions of death. In the gospel of St Thomas, Logion 18 describes an occasion when:

> The disciples said to Jesus, 'Tell us in what way our end will be.' Jesus said, 'Have you therefore discerned the beginning since you seek after the end? For in the Place where beginning is, there will be the end. Happy is he who will stand boldly at the beginning, he shall Know the end, and shall find Life independent of death.'   Ross, 1998

I suspect that what Jesus had to say would not be out of place in the teachings of many different faiths, which lead us inexorably to see death as part of life, as a time of transformation in life and not an ending.

Jesus went on in the Beatitudes to offer a further glimpse, specifically about how an encounter with bereavement, however painful it might be, can also be a blessing. Jesus said, 'Blessed are those who mourn, for they will be comforted' (Matthew 5: 4). His announcement that eternal life dwelt in every person was reinforced by the gift of mourning. How can this be so? Those in the midst of mourning and its agony can hardly be expected to see a blessing there. Amidst often-inexplicable tragedy and suffering, when death arrives in its myriad forms, how on earth can death be seen as a gift? Perhaps in time it can be, but it would seem an impossible perspective to explore when someone is in the midst of bereavement. Perhaps later, when the pain subsides a little, those in helping roles can help towards the resolution of grief by finding in it . . . what? hope, possibility, meaning.

Synthesising a Hindu-Christian perspective, John Martin Sahajananda, a follower of Bede Griffiths, writes that those who mourn may be brought to realise, if they do not already, 'that much of their happiness is a passing happiness that comes from others and is not real happiness that comes from God . . . people who lose their earthly source of happiness may realise its passing nature and so find eternal happiness' (Sahajananda, 2003). Therefore the gift of death can be, paradoxically, not just terrible loss but also the potential for gain, a metanoia of our way of seeing the world that moves us from attachment to only the transient nature of life in this reality, to the possibility of life that is not transient in another realm of being. To see death and loss as a gift, as having potential for more and not just less, can be superhumanly difficult when we are caught up in the midst of it. That is why the presence of wise persons at the time of death can be so profoundly healing through the pain. That is why so many spiritual teachings in many faiths urge us to prepare for death now as part of life.

Henri Nouwen (1997) writes:

> Maybe the death you fear is not simply the death at the end of your present life. Maybe the death at the end of your life won't be so fearful if you can die well now. Yes the real death – the passage from time into eternity, from the transient beauty of this world to the

lasting beauty of the next, from darkness to light – has to be made now. And you do not have to make it alone.

Dying into life does not have to come at the endpoint of our physical existence. Rather, as the words of Jesus, the Buddha and other great teachers cited above suggest, we can awaken now and live our lives even more fully from the resting place in our consciousness where we come to know that 'this is not all there is'. The painful gift of the dead can be an offering in life that points the way to an absolute reality that transcends this one.

CHAPTER 22

GETTING OUT WHEN IT GETS TOO MUCH – THE JOURNEY IS THE GOAL

The road is so beautiful, says the lad.
The road is so hard, says the youth.
The road is so long, says the man.
The old man sits on the roadside to rest.
Sunset colours his beard a reddish gold.
Grass gleams at his feet with evening dew.
A late bird sings unbidden.
Will you remember how long the road was, and how beautiful?

Siddur Lev Chadash (Union of Liberal and Progressive Synagogues, 1995)

GETTING ON AND NEEDING HELP

The personal experience of grief and bereavement in Chapter 21 reinforced for me how our culture seems to really struggle with loss of almost any kind – looks, possessions, health and so on. Tagged on to this are some deep-seated fears around loss of independence. I have vivid memories of an old lady, a neighbour of mine who lived a few doors away when I was ten years old. She had her own home, but we began to see less and less of her, and when she did appear she would hobble to the shops. I offered to help carry her shopping once but she muttered an expletive and lashed out at me with her walking stick. When she died, it was days before someone called to find her lying on the floor in a squalid unkempt home. I learned something then about how some people will never surrender to help no matter how bad it gets.

Despite an ageing population, we live in a culture of accelerating geronto-phobia, full of fear about becoming older, generating a 'particular glorification of youthfulness and an irrational denial of the natural life processes of ageing and dying' (Kimble, 2001). Both individual and social attitudes prevent us from 'age-ing wholly' (Hudson, 2003) seeing old age as an almost entirely negative phenomenon, replete only with decline on all fronts. In a brilliant speech at a recent conference, Rosalie Hudson joined those pushing back the boundaries of the way we think about ageing. After all, the way we think about ageing is just that – thoughts – and thoughts have no power of their own except what we choose to give them. Suppose we start to think of ageing as a time of fulfilment, fruition and reward? Supposing we shift our negative view of dependency into a positive one, enabling new forms of connection with others?

Hudson (2003) writes that:

> *Productivity, technology, lucidity, capacity, independence, autonomy, and the supremacy of individual rights and physical perfection measure the spirit of the age. Rather than a spirited age this seems to be an age without spirit, without heart; an age not conducive to ageing wholly.*

Growing old for many is a dis-spiriting experience when it could be a time of renewal and fulfilment of our spiritual path. Yes, I can see that part of me, down the long tunnel of my fear, that doesn't want to be at end stage of dementia or wheelchair-bound after a stroke. But that view has been nourished by my Western, individualist, rationalist upbringing that sees me as my body and mind, all there is of me. When these go, what's left? If I am just my body and mind, then being independent and autonomous must be the sacred cows I worship. Hudson further comments that:

> *The irony is that we want to uphold autonomy for the elderly at just the time when their condition makes autonomy least attainable, and at a time in life when other human needs – for care, for respect, for meaning – are more pressing. Yet the poverty of our moral discourse is such that we can only offer to those in the last stage of life more autonomy.*

Our near-obsession with autonomy blinds us to other opportunities of ageing and to other connections. I meditate. It is the place and time (paradoxically, spaceless and timeless) where I sit with my Self. Could ageing and any associated disability be not just a time of loss, but a time of gain? If when I am old I do not or cannot move around so much, maybe that is my golden opportunity to go deep into my meditation practice and continue the exploration of that boundless inner world now that my exploration of the outer world is limited?

Could dependence be a transforming power, an opportunity of deepening our connection with each other and with our deepest selves? As Ram Dass points out (2000) in his insights into his own ageing and disability, after a lifetime of helping others he has learned that the shadow of his illness was enlightened by the joy of being in relationship with others where they could express their need to help him. Helping is not a linear one-way relationship from A to B; it is a mutual process, with helper and helped both gaining, as we explored in Chapter 19. Thus 'autonomy' is something of a limited concept at any age, let alone old age. The spirit of old age, if we are to 'age wholly', worships in a different temple, the place of the 'transforming power, or spirit, of *inter*dependence (or heteronomy) over and the prevailing spirit of idealised independence (or autonomy)' (Hudson, 2003). The spirit of old age may be less about needing autonomy, and more about needing each other.

BEING A BURDEN

'I don't want to be a burden.' I can't say I've lost count of the number of times I've heard that from patients: I've heard it so often it's never been worth counting. It's a standard cliché that arises among those who feel they may be too old and/or ill to cope by themselves, or think they may be dying, or those who at some point have given some thought to their own death, which is pretty much all of us. I've heard it most recently from a sick old lady in a nearby bed during a visit to my local hospital. Her body looked, and smelled, in a bad way and relatives arrived one after the other to console and comfort. 'You're not a burden, Mam,' fell on deaf ears.

The current debate around euthanasia has heated up, not least because a House of Lords committee is reviewing the Assisted Dying Bill as I write in late 2004. Whether the law will change or not remains to be seen, but helping somebody to die remains a highly contentious and polarised debate. Professional bodies for healthcare professionals, such as the Royal College of Nursing (RCN) and the British Medical Association (BMA), are under pressure from some of their members to reconsider their current policies, and strong lobbying campaigns are under way. Adverts by pro-'choice' people have appeared in the national media. Various surveys suggest that around 60–70 per cent of nurses are in favour of a change in the law to permit euthanasia, that is, killing people legally (euthanasia sounds so much nicer, doesn't it?). Perhaps the debate, which is as old as the hills, would be a little clearer if we used less euphemism and more direct language.

Some high-profile cases, such as that of Diane Pretty, who in 2004 wanted help to die to end her suffering and the 'burden' she was placing on others because of her motor neurone disease, have added to the media seduction and the call for simplistic solutions. Pictures of suffering people are rarely counterbalanced by the views of those who are patients of palliative-care nurses and doctors, for example, who have a long track record of demonstrating that many forms of suffering (not just physical) can be ameliorated.

One media commentator suggested that he wouldn't allow his dog to suffer in the way we allow some human beings to. This is also a frequently used argument in the pro-euthanasia camp. And it includes the breathtaking assumption that we apply the same rules to animals as we do to people. I am deeply sceptical that such values are a sound basis for making end-of-life decisions.

And the 'being a burden' cry is another assumption that needs to be challenged – for the values around dependency/independency infect our whole culture, as I have suggested above. At almost every level we are given the signal that to be self-caring is good, to need care is bad. Thus the fear of being a burden is often rooted in internalised feelings of low self-worth or the taking on board of cultural norms and views about dependency (see also Chapter 15, and the discussion on positive role models in ageing, especially the significance of 'being' when 'doing' may be inhibited). It's probably true that someone in the midst of deep suffering, such as profound physical pain or disability, is not going to be easily receptive to (or maybe even has the time left for) psychotherapy or spiritual counselling to shift their view of themselves and others on the subject. But in my experience of working with the dying and those who fear they may be dying, this is not impossible, if managed with sensitivity and skill. And experts in palliative care know that people who ask to die in the midst of suffering and dependency are much more circumspect once the suffering, such as pain, is relieved and they are helped to feel less guilty about dependency after all.

In our culture 'dependence' is bad and 'independence' is good. But we are not islands. Independence is an illusion. Our humanity rests upon the connection that we all depend on each other in different ways at different times of our lives. We have need of others when we can't manage alone. But we also have needs to be needed. Our humanity is made real as we connect with each other when the need for help and the need to give help, qualities possessed by all human beings, are brought together. Being with others in their suffering can be one of the most demanding of human experiences, but it can also be one of the most rewarding. And at a simple practical level, if people didn't need help with the relief of their suffering, then nurses and other healthcare workers would be out of a job!

Yet, as I observed in that little encounter in hospital described above, we seem to have no problem with a language to express our disgust (of ourselves) at being a burden, but real difficulty with language to counter it. Giving way to long-held negative values about dependency in ourselves and others is the easy option. It's much tougher to challenge them. I have no problem with the principle that people should be able to choose the timing and manner of their death. The sticking point is one of ensuring that the choice is fully informed. Someone strung out on feelings that they are a burden or that their suffering can never be relieved is psychologically stuck on certain assumptions that may not be true when they are fully explored and healed.

Meanwhile, healthcare staff remain at the forefront of dealing with those whose suffering is so great that they want out by the death route. Killing somebody is not technically, and for some not morally, difficult. Whether those, such as nurses and doctors, who have an ethos of dedication to a life and health enshrined in their professional value systems, should ever be involved at that level with patients – if killing because of suffering becomes legalised is a matter that the professions have not adequately addressed. The two-thirds or so of nurses who think that such killing should be legalised might be more reticent if actually asked to do it.

The tougher path for us is to confront, even in the midst of suffering, the possibility of healing people out of low expectations of relief and the belief being dependent is 'bad'. I wonder if we have the skill, the commitment and even the courage to do that?

TAKING CARE OF DYING – A SPIRITUAL DILEMMA TOO

The discussion on euthanasia has already and inevitably polarised between the fors and againsts. Opinion rubs against opinion, generating more heat than light. Opinions change and are treacherous territory and, likewise, policies based on opinions. It is symptomatic of an unresolved debate that something will inevitably arise to stir the pot of its murky stew once more; in my time long ago as chair of the RCN Ethics Committee, it was the (in)famous Anthony Bland case – a young man left after the Hillsborough tragedy in that tellingly and rather nastily named diagnostic state of PVS (persistent vegetative state). In the struggle to formulate a policy for the RCN in the face of a Gadarene rush towards a simplistic solution being espoused by so many (suffering at death is intolerable and so people should have the 'right' to die and nurses should be prepared to help), the Ethics Committee, RCN Council and a congress debate decided to hold the line. Euthanasia was and should remain illegal.

I think we could have gone further at that time by confronting some difficult questions – the answers to which need to be sought if we are not to repeat history – but first of all we need to be clear about the nature of the debate. It is not just a moral, ethical, social, political, psychological or biological one – for it is all of these and none. It is profoundly rooted in the very essence of what meaning and purpose we bring to our humanity. This is a spiritual problem and spiritual problems require spiritual solutions. Trying to answer the question in terms of 'right' or 'wrong' is a hopelessly dualistic and polarising perspective.

It is not just breadth of opinion needed here (and we can ping-pong endlessly between the extremes) but real depth of understanding, and we might form better laws and policies as a result. So, here I offer my top three of many questions to be faced, but in doing so there is a caveat. The search for truth also requires honesty – honesty about our language. Words like euthanasia and assisted-suicide slip steadily into the realms of euphemism; we are talking about killing people here. Honesty about ourselves is needed, too – picking through the wasteland of our own clichés, prejudices and assumptions. How far is the desire to end the suffering of others contaminated by our need to relieve our own suffering at witnessing it? 'I wouldn't let my dog die like this,' some say. Fine – but do we really equate dogs with human beings, as I suggested above? Those of us who are not actually dying can be rather cocksure about what we would like to happen at the time of death, for others and ourselves; those actually confronting death tend to be much more tentative.

1   What is it to be a person? If we are not clear about what marks out the uniqueness of our humanity, then we cannot be clear about the right action to take in the face of suffering close to the end of life. Do I stop being a person when all those things – my memory, my personality and so on, by which I was once defined – fade away (as in PVS or Alzheimer's, for example)? A (simplistic) biological perspective could answer 'yes' to this. If the brain is no longer working, and the brain is the repository of mind or consciousness, then 'I' no longer exist. The body left behind is indeed just flesh and bone and little else, to be done with as we wish, for it is no longer human. Science has never been able to solve the riddle of consciousness. How can a bunch of neurones, enzymes and the like generate the complexity of a personality or explain our response to a production of a Beethoven symphony, a painting by Gaugin or a poem by Eliot? Other traditions would suggest that consciousness is not just in the body, but that the body is in consciousness. Who I am is infinitely greater than the mere collocation of atoms that makes up my physical body and its processes. Millennia of human experience, equally valid in my view to much of modern research methods, suggest that people not only believe but know, through direct experience, that we do not end at our skin.

2   What is suffering? 'Suffering is,' said the Buddha. He saw it from the grand perspective of his enlightened state, as the product of the mind's interminable attachment to its fears, needs and desires. The seductive view that all suffering can be avoided is a fairly recent phenomenon, fuelled by Western scientific advances and the culture of eternal youth – the marketing of the possibility of a perfect lifestyle, body, health, home, garden, etc. Viewed from this standpoint suffering is not only resolvable but also meaningless. Yet other perspectives might see it differently. 'Suffering is grace,' from the Hindu-influenced Ram Dass (2002), means shifting us out of our limiting view of ourselves into a deeper connection with a deeper reality. Jesus spoke of 'metanoia' – using the suffering of this life and the things that have happened to us in the past as an opportunity to 'transform' ourselves (Ross, 1998) and, in this case, approach God ever more closely. Suffering, from these perspectives, has meaning, purpose and

possibility. Others would see suffering and how you respond to it as affecting your next incarnation – the Hindu believes that where your consciousness is at the time of death affects where you go next. Gandhi, as the gunshot hit, famously cried out 'Ram' (God) – for to be with God in your mind at the point of death, unclouded by fear or the mist of drugs, is considered profoundly significant in spiritual evolution. The relief of suffering is furthermore a co-creative process (it does, after all, provide jobs for healthcare practitioners!) for we are drawn into it too. It can indeed be a tall order to see suffering as purposeful when you are in the middle of it. However, the frontier work of people like Dame Cicely Saunders and the ensuing hospice and palliative-care movement, and truly holistic approaches such as that of the Bristol Cancer Help Centre, offer us practical solutions. Suffering at the end of life is neither meaningless nor inevitable. More imaginative approaches than limited drug regimes, for example, can make a reality of metanoia for all of us. Suffering can be transcended; we can be healed even while dying.

3   Is participating in euthanasia the work of established professionals such as doctors or nurses? If the role of the practitioner is about the relief of suffering, and its prime directive is just that, then the logical conclusion is that this might include helping people to 'top' themselves when the suffering becomes unbearable. Given that we have explored all the avenues – suggested therapy if the patient is depressed or feeling worthless, tried all the drugs, or given up on the lavender-oil massage, then maybe there is a case for helping to see people off when they no longer want to stay on. On the other hand, is this too risky? A profession dedicated to caring for others, the relief of suffering and the importance of life might find itself caught up in a schizoid dilemma if it also embraces killing people, however kindly we express it or carry it out. If the law changes to permit euthanasia and assisted suicide (and countries that have tried it have run into huge problems), can a patient really have confidence in a nurse or doctor who cares but may also kill? Would the conflicting signals be untenable for them and for us, even if killing is part of caring? Would such a philosophical and practical embrace by carers fundamentally change the nature of the patient–helper relationship? Or perhaps a new occupation would have to emerge, a sort of Death Care Assistant, suitably trained, ready and willing when called, or maybe a consultant nurse specialising in thanatology. We have them now, outside the law. They are called relatives, or the Jack Kevorkians or the hidden nurses and doctors in quiet collusion, skirting the very edges of professional and legal boundaries.

The territory of euthanasia is fraught with pitfalls and it is a landscape we seem destined to be trapped in until we get a little more honesty in our language and seek some answers to some bigger truths, going beyond the siren calls of the absolutes of 'rights' and 'choice'.

THE LAST GASP OF THE EGO

Whatever decisions healthcare practitioners make around the time of death, and no matter how we struggle with the moral and ethical issues, some people have a knack of bypassing the system completely and make a decision to end their suffering, whatever its form, by killing themselves. I remember the first 'overdose' I encountered. He was a young man, admitted to Foulds' Ward at Bury General Hospital. I trained there donkey's years ago and they've probably flattened it now. Student nurses made up a sizeable part of the workforce in those days, and as a bumbling first-year I was profoundly impressed by the depth of knowledge of a rather aloof third-year, especially on the theme of suicide. She'd read a book about it.

'It's just a cry for help,' she said and I remember the particular curl of eyebrow and lip as she said it. It was the face of a woman who knew a thing or two, or thought she did. In middle age I find myself certain only of being uncomfortable with such certainty. I was impressed at the time, but I looked at her and at the pale young man in his obvious and abject misery and I thought, 'Well, I can see the crying – but where's the help?'

The 'cry for help' cliché invades all manner of judgements about people's difficulties, from violent fathers to that spurious 'diagnosis' of Münchhausen's by proxy. Oh, the attempted suicide is indeed a cry from the voiceless, sometimes, a response to a deep unarticulated pain within the wounded ego, the soul's implacable gaoler, desperate to be reconciled yet unable to say how. Sometimes, too, it's a neat diagnosis that avoids individuals' taking responsibility for their own failings or (in)ability to address the tough events of life.

My mother would have made an interesting nurse at such moments. The stoicism and resilience that were the products of English working-class life between the Wall Street Crash and World War II, compounded by full-time parenting in pre-NHS days, could seem harsh in the face of another's suffering. Had she been a nurse (unschooled and a full-time mum, she never got past being a cleaning lady), she would have belonged very much to the 'pull yourself together' school – 'Pull yourself together, don't you realise there's people out there far worse off than you are?'

> 'But I don't want the veg, mum.'
> 'Eat it, there's kids starving in Africa, be glad of it.'
> 'Then send it to 'em.'
> Slap!

I suspect that the likes of those deeply politically incorrect thoughts of my mother lurk around in the dark recesses of many of us – the little value-judgements that dare not speak their name.

Some say it takes courage to kill yourself (Lott, 2004). I was once in a place in my life where my own death seemed the only way to be free of the agony, but I never was tough enough to actually do it. Paradoxically, killing oneself has a cowardice dimension too – a quick escape from suffering rather than facing it. It also has an essentially selfish dimension as well – we may rationalise it and convince ourselves that the world would be better off without us, but my experience of families who have lost someone to suicide is that a pain is created that lasts for ever. They loved me enough to leave and spare my suffering, but did they not love me enough to stay and keep loving me, to spare me the greater suffering of their loss?

I have encountered some people in my life, and not always in my professional capacity, whose inner pain is so searing and bottomless that death seems the only way out. Last year, a sweet woman I know killed herself. She had been wrestling with her demons for 20 years and she'd had enough. When our ego is bereft, for whatever reason, of that deep sense of connection with the world or with the love of God (however you see it), and sees nothing but the void, one can see why we might want out. When the abyss not only opens before you, but also becomes you, then maybe all the last power you have is to remove yourself from this reality.

I remember a poem at school, one of those you were *made* to learn (Tennyson's 'The Revenge'), and the words remain with me to this day. 'At Flores on the Azores, Sir Richard Grenville lay . . .' and the verse unfolds to tell of the noble admiral's entrapment. Rather than submit, he sinks his own ship, 'Sink me the ship master gunner, sink her, split her in twain.' Those lines have stuck in my brain from all those years ago . . . and they surfaced when I learned of my friend's self-hanging. Our ego needs power; it is its raison d'être. But disconnected from a deeper level of existence – from soul, from God, from the Absolute or the immortal higher Self – the ego is cut adrift with ships of despair all around and seemingly no way out but down. This is no cry for help. This is spiritual collapse and our mental health services seem hopelessly ill-equipped to deal with it. The antidepressants, the psychotherapies in all their forms, may stay the executioner's hand for a while, but he will lurk forever in the background until the person can come home to their preciousness and their value in the greater realm of being.

Stripped of its power and control – of life, against pain – the pressing of the self-destruct button is paradoxically the last gesture of the ego; the power to destroy itself is the only power it has left.

CHAPTER 23
EXPLORING THE LANDSCAPE OF THE SOUL

We join spokes together in a wheel,
But it is the centre hole that makes the wagon move.
We shape clay into a pot,
But it is the emptiness inside that holds whatever we want.
We hammer wood for a house,
But it is the inner space that makes it liveable.
We work with being,
But not being is what we use.

Tao Te Ching (Streep, 1994)

A MOMENT OF SPIRITUAL CARE IN ACTION

His English was poor and little was known of his background except that he was Moslem. A stranger in the strange land of hospital, his fear and panic were rising in parallel with the pain. His voice reached screaming pitch and nurses and doctors gathered. Attempts to calm him veered between the pointless ('Please be quiet, you're disturbing the other patients') to the judgemental and perhaps downright racist ('He's just after attention' and 'Some of them do have lower pain thresholds').

The staff were probably doing their best, but their understanding was wide of the mark, an interpreter could not be found and the man was sinking deeper into the stew of terror in this alienating landscape. One care assistant, quieter than the rest, had been holding back. She felt she had something to help but had not the courage to use it. Her trepidation was finally overcome by frustration and anger at the comments of her colleagues. She pushed the others to one side, called the patient by name and clearly and firmly said 'La illa Ha illa Allah'. The effect was instant. The patient grasped the assistant's hand and an air of calm enveloped them as they both simply looked each other in the eye. No further words could be said or were necessary. The man had just been given something to put him at peace, better than anything drawn up in the nearby syringes. In the twinkling of an eye, he had been shown that he was understood and accepted, he was not alone, he was connected.

My friend had come to be the butt of a few jokes among her colleagues. She had felt the limitations of her ability to meet the spiritual needs of patients and had decided to follow a course in interfaith ministry. She was learning fast that ministering to patients' spiritual needs is not about performing rituals with them, but coming to understand their belief systems so that she could say and do the right thing at the right time. It is about being open and available to people when they ask you those difficult questions about the meaning of suffering, or listening to their fear and unhappiness when they are feeling that their God is not with them or when they feel cut adrift and afraid in the midst of suffering. Ministry for her had come to include answering questions honestly when those tentative remarks came from her colleagues. There is no need for proselytising; just being her honest integruous self is all that is needed when people want to talk about God, the Absolute, the meaning of life or whatever (we all do at some point and, as her colleagues' reactions illustrated, public embarrassment or jocularity often hides private interest).

Studying the interfaith course had deepened her understanding of the different faiths – vital if she was to get away from 'handover syndrome': finding out the patient's religion, then handing the rest of the problem over to the nearest chaplain.

Meeting the spiritual needs of patients is everybody's business, yet the evidence suggests that we still lack both the personal and professional capacity to deal with spiritual matters. Interfaith studies (Wright & Sayre Adams, 2000; Holden, 2002a) seem to be one way forward, but as yet our educational programmes remain sadly lacking in this area. We still tend to reduce the teaching of the faith aspects of nursing to checking out the patients' dietary needs or the traditions about bodily contact. This superficial approach ignores the depth of meaning that faith, of whatever sort, can bring to patients and ourselves – it avoids the potential of a vibrant spiritual assessment. Perhaps most worryingly, it dances around the difficulty that spiritual care cannot be fully realised unless carers have themselves explored and enriched their understanding of their own spiritual needs, knowledge, prejudices, wounds and motives. Thus, much of the profession remains stuck in either avoiding spiritual care altogether or thinking that we can teach spiritual care as some kind of object 'out there', rather than something that is deeply connected within ourselves. Understanding spirituality is not an intellectual exercise: it is a lived experience.

My friend showed great courage with her patient that day and the effect was a startling transformation in his response. It was not that she said what are probably the most potent words in Islam (the translation is 'There is no god but

God'), rather the way that she said it. In the midst of a crisis with things getting out of hand and a patient's suffering accelerating, her knowing what would
matter to this man shone through. The words, in a language he could comprehend, created an instant de-alienating effect. His faith was made real by the
acknowledgement and presence of someone who could break through the
language barrier to that place beyond words where we know we are safe
because we are in the hands of someone who understands.

It could have been any faith and any carer, but it took not just knowledge
about the faith; it also took the carer's knowing of herself to be able to carry
it off.

SPIRITUAL ASSESSMENT?

There doesn't seem to be a branch of health care that has not, as David Stoter
(1995) has noted, relegated spiritual care to a footnote on the patient's religion
in the case notes. I've had cause to visit over a score of healthcare settings in
recent months, yet none had developed spiritual assessment approaches and
indeed, as Stoter has suggested, most carers remain perplexed and lacking in
confidence in anything to do with spirituality. A recent study with albeit a small
sample size (77 nurses) bears out the continuing uncertainty that many nurses
feel about spirituality in patient care (Nathan, 2000). In this research a majority of nurses clearly saw the need for spiritual support for their clients, but they
also lacked know-how about how to do so, and their education in the subject
was often sorely lacking.

Some recent publications are addressing this issue, but many textbooks still
skirt around it, or confusingly focus on religious rituals and customs instead of
addressing spiritual matters, for example how to deal with the hygiene needs
of an Islamic patient rather than understand what their faith means to them and
the way they deal with a health crisis.

McSherry (2000) provides a useful guide to the deeper understanding of
spirituality and the implications for nurses, especially from a Judaeo-Christian
perspective. There are many helpful self-assessment questions in this work, so
it's not just a practical guide but an educational tool too. Guidelines for assessing patients' spiritual needs include appropriate questions to be asked (such as
'Is prayer helpful to you? What happens when you pray? And so on). McSherry also urges us not only to choose the right questions, but also to decide *when*
to ask them.

Engel et al. (2000) have documented ways in which doctors and others can
take a spiritual history, by probing sensitively into a patient's perceptions of
their spiritual needs. This begins with questions about religious and spiritual
practices ('Do you belong to any spiritual or religious community?') and then

moves on to look at ways of giving specific support ('What aspects of your religion/spirituality would you like me to keep in mind as I care for you?'). Dossey (1996) has looked at ways in which we can not only assess the patient's needs, but also participate appropriately, such as asking the patient if they mind being prayed for by the doctor. There are some adventurous ways of joining patients to meet their spiritual needs here, but it is a minefield of potential misunderstandings and mistakes – especially if carers allow their own prejudices and religious enthusiasms to get in the way.

Burkhardt and Jacobsen (2000) offer some of the best insights and ways of helping and it's a text I often turn to for advice. There are clear suggestions on questions to be asked of patients and when to ask them – everything from 'Do you meditate?' to 'How do you feel about yourself right now?' A self-assessment scale for patients enables them to rate their feelings on a range of issues from 'My life has meaning and purpose' to 'My inner strength is related to belief in a higher power or supreme being', and from 'There is fulfilment in my life' to 'Reconciling relationships is important to me'.

Practical guidance like this is providing the foundation for healthcare practitioners to get involved appropriately and safely in meeting the spiritual needs of patients. It is still, however, uncertain territory, while so many carers remain ill-educated in best practice. As suggested in Chapter 11, some moves are under way to give practitioners help in how to assess and deliver spiritual care, but much work remains to be done.

For example, the NHS in Scotland produced a groundbreaking document (in NHS terms at least) providing guidance on the development of spiritual care services in the Scottish NHS (NHS Scotland, 2002). It sought, among other things, to make distinctions between spiritual and religious care (see Chapter 1) and how spiritual care services can be best delivered in a multi-faith society. It acknowledged, while suggesting that chaplaincy should be focused in 'Departments of Spiritual and Religious Care', that this type of care was delivered by a very broad range of people, both formally and informally. And, crucially, while seeing spiritual and religious care as fundamental to NHS objectives, it affirmed that it needs 'the distinctive contribution of caregivers who are trained in spiritual and religious care and have time to give it'.

The report is inclusive and embracing of interfaith perspectives and, dare I say it, for a government product, surprisingly radical, forward-thinking and very practical in the options it proposes. The document did not pretend to have all the answers and many of the suggestions were contentious, but it was interesting to see that even government-level policymaking was now recognising that spiritual care is everyone's business; it's not just for the chaplain or the specialist nurse with a degree in theology. The thorny question is to make sure that the right sort of holistic support is given by the right people with the right skills and knowledge (see Chapter 11).

And to reiterate a caution about that much-abused word 'holism'. Holistic care is *not* about adding spiritual care to physical, social and mental care. Holism in its true sense originated in the new physics community to describe the evidence of the way in which everything that appears to be separate is actually connected (this was no news to mystics!). Holism suggests that we are part of all that is and any boundaries are illusory. An acceptance of holism in the field of health care has enormous implications for the way we see ourselves and work with patients and our colleagues. Spirituality in this concept is not an add-on, but an integral part of the whole; there is nothing that is not spiritual. Dualism (me patient – you nurse; me subject – you God) does not exist in a holistic universe except in our perceptions. In a holistic reality there is no separation – and that implies a huge shift of approach to the way we deliver spiritual care.

Furthermore, it is not enough to think of spirituality as 'a thing out there', something we deliver to patients like drugs through an IV line. Spirituality is 'in here' in each of us as carers. Consideration for the spiritual needs of others is intimately bound up with meeting our own spiritual needs. When nurses and others are well-grounded in their own spiritual wellbeing, they are infinitely more available to meet the needs of others (Wright & Sayre-Adams, 2000). Any policy developments for patients must be tied in with meeting the spiritual needs of staff. The two go hand in hand.

Some may find that they can explore their spiritual needs through their current religious frameworks, others on such programmes I have discussed above, yet others through a commitment to spiritual voyaging across the vast ocean of opportunities available. One starting point is for practitioners to look at the spiritual assessment tools such as those listed above, and try answering the questions before they even attempt to work with patients on these themes. In the current spiritual supermarket, there is no shortage of ways open to us to explore spirituality, bearing in mind the cautions I have explored in Chapters 9 and 11.

When I first began to write about spiritual matters in health care, a lecturer colleague told me not to! Looking at so many other innovations in health care, especially on ways of documenting things, he felt we would just make a mess of it again and reduce what should be a finely tuned part of care into a rote and checklist ritual. 'Look at what happened with the nursing process,' he said. 'Nurses will just cock it up, by reducing it to a list of questions and you'll end up with some nurse casting out devils instead of giving the Warfarin.' He was joking, I hope, but a recent report in the popular press of a nurse trying to exorcise a sick patient made me realise he could be all too serious. Do we stay away from this territory because we risk a few nurses or other carers making a hash of it, or is this an as-yet little-explored frontier where, with some knowledge and skill, we could bring a real enhancement to people's wellbeing?

IF YOU NEED TO ASK – SHOULD YOU?

As we explore the educational options for healthcare staff in spiritual care, I can't quite get rid of one final niggle that lies at the back of my mind. I'm reminded of a time long ago when my dad was out on the razzle with his mates or working on nights, my mum and I would go shopping rather than sit at home on our own. On the purple and cream 36 bus we'd head for Bolton, the big city to me then, and wander round the streets gazing into the brightly lit shop windows. If mum was feeling a bit flush, we'd have the luxury of a Walsh's pasty (are you still there Mr Walsh?) before heading for the bus home. We never actually went in the shops because they were all closed. If my mum had been a nurse, she would have probably joined an AIDS campaign for safe sex – she knew all about prevention, in this case 'safe shopping'. The knack, of course, was to head for the shops in the evening after closing time – that way you could enjoy window shopping, safe in the knowledge that the family finances would be unchallenged.

I distinctly remember one occasion when my mum admired a particularly fine coat in the window at the Co-op. There was no price on it. The longing look in my mum's eyes said it all. In my naivety, having no grasp at that age of what it was to be 'poor', I suggested we could come back in the day and buy it. 'How much does it cost, mum?' 'I don't know,' she replied, 'but you can be sure if you have to ask you can't afford it.' Her wisdom escaped me then and, anyway, 'Let's go for a pasty' was an easy distractor.

For some reason this childhood memory of a cold winter night in Bolton came to mind at a recent spirituality and health conference. Erudite papers were presented and workshops convened on the best examples of carrying out spiritual assessment by healthcare professionals. An assortment of questionnaires and guidelines was on offer, mirroring the proliferation of such examples in the nursing and other literature. Yet amidst the helpful debate, that memory of my mum chattered away at my shoulder like some spiritual Jimminy Cricket.

I recall the advent of the 'nursing process' to the UK that I mentioned above, and the flood of nursing assessment tools that appeared in the literature, the conferences organised on the theme in the mid-1980s and not a few books published either, among which, for my sins, I must include myself! Some years later, my partner was admitted to hospital. Flat on his back and in agonising pain, he watched as the nurse entered and announced that she had come to 'do the nursing process'. I sat quietly in the background as the nurse, rote-like, went through the questionnaire and pursued lines like 'Has this condition made any difference to your sex life?' Caught between hysterics and despair, I had to leave the room.

There may be some truth in the view that if you need to ask, it's beyond your reach. If you need some form of questionnaire guidance, then you should not be doing it. The encouragement from all quarters, not least recent Health Department guidelines, for those other than chaplains to get involved in assessing spiritual needs is at one level encouraging, at another level scary. Lots of spiritual assessment tools are now available to us and I suspect work is being done on developing even more here and there across the country. But hang on a minute. Perhaps spiritual needs do not lend themselves easily to objective questionnaires and, more importantly, the skills needed to 'find out' demand that the enquirers are themselves spiritually 'awake'.

I have a theory that the capacity to enquire into and deliver spiritual care (and its nature *is* different from, say, psychological or physical support) is directly proportional to the caregiver's spiritual awareness. A person who has explored and rests comfortably in their own spirituality, and who has become a reasonably healed and well-rounded human being, is well placed to ask the right questions and make the right, flexible and sensitive approach – assessment tools are then nothing more than aides-mémoire, if they are needed at all. Unleashing nurses and other carers on patients who have the theory but who have not had the (life) experience fills me with doubt and perhaps a degree of dread. I can see it all now: patient arrives on the ward in pain and with a crushed pelvis as a result of a car accident; in agony in bed, they will be asked by some carer, 'How has this injury affected your spirituality?' Then, on the treatment sheet will appear, 'Prayers TDS and miracles nocte.' Please tell me this won't happen. Please!

The colleague I described at the beginning of this chapter seems to have got the right approach: a combination of intuition, experience, wisdom, knowledge and maturity would seem to offer the best safeguards for patients when carers decide to give spiritual help.

For further information on interfaith education contact:
The Interfaith Seminary,
Mulberry House,
583 Fulham Road,
London SW6 5UA
Tel: 020 7471 1889

CHAPTER 24
PRACTICE MAKES PERFECT

I believe in advaita, I believe in the essential unity of all that lives. Therefore I believe that if one person gains spiritually the whole world gains, and if one person falls, the world falls to that extent.

Gandhi (1924)

IT'S LOVE NOT FEAR

Spirituality doesn't have to be god- (or goddess-) centred, as I have often mentioned in this book. But for most people it is, and all the major faiths hold great store by beliefs about compassionate action to relieve the suffering of others.

Yet, as I have suggested, there are risks to patients if we use our version of God to make a patient's suffering worse (e.g. through being judgemental or proselytising). Likewise, ignoring God completely or assuming that the chaplain will take over misses out an essential element of the healing process for those whose world is theocentric. Finding a healthy balance can be difficult and there need to be some safeguards in place in addition to the rules set out in our code of conduct.

Recently, I witnessed a hellfire Christian condemning a homosexual bishop in particular and homosexuals in general. I just sat there and thought, 'That's not the God I know!' So what is the nature of the God you know?

The atheist doesn't recognise a supernatural deity, so for them the issue doesn't enter the equation. However, this can produce problems in itself, which I will touch on later. For the majority who have some kind of deity, it matters very much how we relate to that being, because that relationship fundamentally affects the way we interact with other human beings. The religious values we derive from or project onto our God underpin how we are with other people. It is worth recalling the words of Miranda Holden (2002a) (cited earlier):

Consciously or unconsciously, if your deepest perception of God is fearful, judgmental, conditional or punishing, you will tend to be judgmental, conditional, fearful, and punishing with yourself . . . Your primal relationship to your God determines how you think of yourself. Unconsciously you project this dynamic onto everyone and everything. Holding onto a fearful image of God is not a good recipe for a happy life.

Curiously, if we look at words like 'suffering', 'fear', 'punish', 'danger' and 'condemn' in some important holy books (such as the Bible, the Qur'an, the Dhammapada, the Upanishads, the Tao te Ching, the Guru Granth Sahib), they appear dozens of times. But words like 'love', 'forgiveness', 'heal' and 'help' outnumber them many times over. In part this fearful God is often a distortion of the way we have been introduced to religion or to early childhood experience of authority figures, be they religious, social or parental. The personal misery this causes would be bad enough, but unfortunately we tend to project our shadow side outwards, as was illustrated in Chapters 10 and 11. As a result, individually and collectively, we can unleash some tremendously destructive forces – from shaming and blaming others to terrible mass atrocities.

Religion often gets condemned for the slaughter conducted in its name. But interestingly, as the religious historian Karen Armstrong has pointed out (Armstrong, 2001), this destructiveness pales against the holocausts of the post-God regimes. In the nineteenth-century age of Darwinism, Nietzsche famously declared that 'God is dead', believing that humanity was now free from dependency on a deity and could fulfil its destiny without the chains of reliance upon supernatural intervention – a view echoed by influential modern Darwinists and atheists such as Richard Dawkins. Sartre, who acknowledged the 'God-shaped hole in modern consciousness' still saw it as a human duty to reject deities, which negated our freedom (Armstrong, 2001). The death of God is indeed liberating to some. However, it is curious that after Nietzsche's God died, the twentieth century saw the unleashing of human nihilism on an unparalleled scale – from the mass slaughters of Armenia and Rwanda, through two world wars, to revolutionary upheaval in Russia, China and Cambodia and so on. Armstrong also reminds us of the words of Chesterton that 'When people cease to believe in God, they don't believe in nothing but will believe in anything.' Atheism, too, can have its shadow side. Whether atheist or theist, when we do not resolve that shadow in ourselves, our belief systems can become the vehicle for inflicting harm on others.

CHECKING OUT OUR EXPERIENCES

Let me briefly mention a couple of examples. The press recently has carried reports about two murderers in the US: one a Mormon, who believed that

God had told him to kill his sister-in-law and niece; another an anti-abortionist, who believed that God and the Bible authorised him to kill a doctor (and his bodyguard) who carried out abortions. Most of us at some time have experienced a mystical communion with the Absolute, an 'inner voice' or profound revelation – be it for a few seconds or perhaps a lifetime (Maxwell & Tschudin, 1996) – as the mystics do. But sorting out the real numinous experience from the false prompting of the shadow side of our egos can be a tricky business. One thing that the religions should do, but often fail at, is provide the monitoring and mentoring of the religious seeker to allow them to safely explore their religious experience and sort out the false from the true.

Hence our mental hospitals are full of people who are having a spiritual crisis but are labelled as psychotic or deluded. Hence people go about committing terrible crimes in God's name or, as in the case of some healthcare practitioners I have encountered, become judgemental or excluding of patients because they do not fit with their godly view, despite professional rules that this is beyond the pale. Spiritual direction, for example from a pastor or priest, should be providing a challenge to the distortions of truth. But this can be difficult if the belief system and those who serve it have themselves not accomplished the emotional/ego work that is necessary to deal with their own 'demons'. Fearful religious leaders rooted in a fearful God can be a frighteningly destructive force, fostering the same shadow in their followers.

Exploring our belief systems is often one of the toughest things we can do, for we stick like glue to them when challenged, if we are influenced by fear. The individual who feels varying degrees of unworthiness, vulnerability and low self-esteem will often mask these shadows by adhering rigidly to a particular belief system – it is a way of being safe, of exercising control in what is perceived to be an unsafe and out-of-control world. So, taking the premise from *A Course in Miracles* (Anon., 1975) that 'God is not fear but love' we have a basis for checking out our religious beliefs and experiences. The experience of Ultimate Reality, whatever we perceive that to be, whether it be some form of deity, pure consciousness or highest human values, should:

- be expansive rather than contracting – the experience leads us to be more present, more available, more loving and more functional in the world, and less angry, threatened, hateful or fearful
- be entirely loving, increasing our capacity to love and be compassionate to others, without the desire to harm ourselves or others
- enable us to be more forgiving, accepting, inclusive and embracing of others, not judgemental, shaming, punishing or exclusive
- deepen our capacity for discernment rather than judgementalism – being more able to sort out the true from the false, the good from the bad, the harmful from the harmless and the important from the trivial

- encourage a sense of trust in ourselves, others and the Absolute that enables us to work collaboratively
- foster humility and the possibility that we are not always right, that we do not always have to be in control and that having our beliefs tested and challenged need not be threatening.

An increasing body of evidence, as I have discussed, is pointing to more involvement by healthcare staff in spiritual care. This cannot be done safely without exploration and testing of our own spiritual values and practices (against, for example, the criteria I have suggested above). How we can sort out the wheat from the chaff with more certainty is no mean challenge.

STAYING ON TRACK

There are both benefits and drawbacks of the spiritual quest and the acceptance or otherwise of some sort of Absolute Reality or Source of All. The spiritual search is not without attendant risks, as Mariana Caplan (1999; 2002) has succinctly pointed out. False gurus and charlatans there are aplenty and the tricks of our own egos are legion. We can easily be led astray by the seductive promises of others or by our own desire not to have our long-cherished perceptions of ourselves challenged or changed. In our efforts to reach a blissful state and stay there, we can find ourselves sidetracked into spiritual practices where we seek only comfort and not disturbance, avoidance of the suffering of the human condition and not the embracing of it. All the great spiritual traditions agree that if there is any point to spiritual practice, it is not to plunge us into a blissed-out state divorced from ordinary humanity; rather we are called ever more deeply into the human experience. Yet our spiritual practice enables us to do so from a different place within ourselves. We participate in the world more fully, embracing all the richness of its joys and sorrows, yet we do so from that place of witness within ourselves that comes to know that we are infinitely more than flesh and blood, that we do not end at our skin. Thus, as one spiritual teacher I met (Jean Shenoda Bolen) reminded me, we come to realise that we are not just human beings having a spiritual experience, but spiritual beings having a human experience.

Spiritual work is no place for the faint-hearted. It's tough work of a lifelong commitment, so it's easy to see why many would prefer to lead lives of denial or self-indulgence. I've lost count of the number of times I've been off to a meditation session, course or retreat in some lovely gathering or site, and returned to 'ordinary reality' feeling open and loving and compassionate – only to lose it rapidly when somebody cuts me up on the motorway! As one nurse, who has been in retreat this week at the Foundation, said to me this morning before I wrote this – 'It's lovely being here and finding what I've been looking for – but how do I keep it going when I get back to house and job and kids?' Part of the solution to this conundrum is, of course, letting go of the desire or expectation of staying blissful, or even that this is a goal of spiritual practice.

First of all, pursue your search in community. Find a group or groups of fellow seekers with whom you can share your experiences and knowledge, meditate or pray together or whatever your spiritual practices are. The established religions offer this (or they are supposed to), but it is possible to find your 'tribe' by other means. I know a group of meditators locally who are from all religious backgrounds and none, yet they meet regularly to support, encourage, question and learn from one another. The community should be like that. If the group is aggressive, controlling, dogmatic or punishing (just like some spiritual teachers), then find the nearest exit.

Second, develop a spiritual practice or practices that give you the time, space and encouragement to commit yourself to your inner work. For me that takes the form of regular episodes of meditation and prayer during the day, spending time in nature, regular t'ai chi and so on. The list of potential spiritual practices is enormous and some may be more obvious than we realise, such as our work or relationships. Deepen your knowledge and skills in one or more of these that work for you. This requires commitment and overcoming the tendency to drop something because it's difficult or doesn't give us what we want. It is right that we should be discerning about what nourishes us, but this also needs to be balanced with the recognition that some spiritual practices are meant to be tough and demand staying power if we are truly to awaken with them.

Third, healthcare workers are used to writing care plans or prescribing treatments. How about writing a spiritual care plan for yourself – embracing your commitment to your practices and how you will take care of yourself physically, mentally, emotionally, socially and spiritually? For me this has included, apart from my specific practices, a commitment to my physical wellbeing by being careful (mostly!) with what I eat and drink, for example I ensure that I have some time each year in silence and solitude and have created spaces in my home and garden dedicated to stillness and contemplation. I know a doctor in a full household who has set up a shelf in her bedroom – in effect an altar – replete with inspiring literature, pictures, flowers and so on. Everyone knows that when Mum is spending her 15 minutes a day in that corner, she is not to be interrupted.

Fourth, seek out literature and the arts that nourish your spiritual quest. There is much inspiring New Age spiritual literature available (and here there is an exercise in discernment, for much of it is also trashy), but established faiths, too, have their tried and tested holy books. Poetry and other literature, music, dance and art can also be deep sources of inspiration and strength.

Fifth, find one or more trusted guides, coaches, gurus or counsellors who can support and challenge you in your spiritual life. This is not work that can be done alone, nor should it be. A trusted guide and a shared community (see above) is essential to help us persist when things get tough (and they will!) and to help us find our way through the risks of false prophets, distorted thinking or confusing experiences. Spiritual direction or counselling takes great skill and experience and it can be hard to find people you can trust. Such persons can often be found in the established faiths, but as I have said before in this book, having a dog collar or other holy vestment is no guarantee of deep and compassionate spirituality. Likewise, those who lay claim to be free of the bounds of any particular faith can be equally prone to judgementalism and power trips. See Chapter 10 for more thoughts on finding your guide or coach.

Meanwhile, it's worth remembering that developing your spiritual practice need not be a joyless labour of abnegation and self-punishment. It should be essentially challenging, but ultimately joyfully so. It's important to be willing to do the work, but at the same time to be easy on yourself and not get into a place of 'If it ain't hurting, it ain't working.' We need to find a balance between allowing ourselves to be stretched spiritually, yet developing our spiritual care plan according to our opportunities, abilities and other life commitments. Setting goals of, say, two hours of meditation a day or an annual fortnight of retreat can be impossible with a houseful of kids and other responsibilities. Tailoring our spiritual practice to the commitments of ordinary life does not mean that we have to make compromises – it's quality rather than quantity of commitment that counts. Sometimes less is more. Indeed our everyday relationships and work, as I have suggested, might provide opportunities as spiritual practices in themselves – all we have to do is wake up to them.

RIGHT UNDER YOUR NOSE (1)

A reader of my *Nursing Standard* series said to me, 'It's OK for you at your age and your time of life.' (I took a deep breath at this point and uttered a brief inner prayer to let go of my murderous thoughts!) 'Your kids are grown up, you've done what you wanted in your career. Me, I've got the house to sort out, my degree work, the kids to get to school, my husband to keep happy .. . I've no time for this spiritual stuff like you.'

On the contrary, it may be that the very ordinary stuff of our lives can be turned to deepening our awareness of who we are and how we participate in all that is. All that needs to shift is our awareness of this possibility.

One such spiritual path is the path of our everyday relationships. If spiritual practice takes us ever more deeply into truth and love, then there is no better place to find them than, as Shantanand Saraswati (cited in Boux, 1999) observes, in the relationships we have now:

> One has to discover the source which is love and all relationships by which all things have their being. Mother, father, sister, brother, colleague and all relationships have some aspect of love. One needs to learn and respond naturally to these relationships in their power and sense. Simple and truthful relation is all we need to maintain.

Walsch (1995) writes:

> You have nothing to learn about relationships, you have only to demonstrate what you already know. There is a way to be happy in relationships and that is to use relationships for their intended purpose . . . relationships are constantly challenging; constantly calling you to create, express, and experience higher and higher aspects of yourself, grander and grander visions of yourself, ever more magnificent versions of yourself. Nowhere can you do this more immediately, impact fully and immaculately than in relationships. In fact, without relationships, you cannot do it at all.

Relationships provide us with the milieu to discover who we are by providing all the possible emotional experiences by which we can both learn and expand our consciousness. Newman (1986), indeed, has described health as 'expanding consciousness'. In relationships we often see it as possible to find completeness with another It might be more appropriate to see relationships as an opportunity for us to express our completeness.

Our everyday relationships can be part of our spiritual discipline if we approach them consciously as the testbed for our spiritual awakening. What is the point of learning of love and compassion, of connectedness with the Divine, the Absolute or the Universal Consciousness or our deeper purpose in life, whatever we perceive these to be, if we cannot bring that into our daily lives? Relationships provide us with the opportunity to 'walk our talk' – put into practice what we preach about spirituality.

Jones (1996) notes that our relationships do not have to be in a state of constant connectedness and harmony:

> Through the process of joining and separating again and again we learn to establish our identity in relation to others. The ebb and flow of closeness and distance maintains the dynamic balance between autonomy and connection. Times of separation undergird our individuality; times of connection keep us related to those around us.

In the West, we tend to expect that the only measure for a successful relationship is one of eternal bliss and happiness. If it is not working, then maybe we should move on to the next one. 'One likes to believe that any trouble in a relationship is caused by outside circumstances, or the other partner. If only he or she would change, how perfect life would be!' note Pierrakos and Saly (1993). 'Yet in the landscape of our souls the lower self and its effects also need to be discovered. Without facing what we least like about ourselves, we cannot understand why we do not have a well-working relationship, let alone make significant change.' And relationship is about our connection not just with other people, but also in ourselves, for much of spiritual work is a gradual exploration and letting-go of ego identities.

We live by roles and identities, but if part of your identity has to be kept under wraps because the rest of the world disapproves of it, then that can be a real challenge to living. One example concerns that of a young male friend of mine, Chris (not his real name), who learned that to be gay means that one has passed through the baptism of fire that 'coming out' can sometimes be. (Although I am referring to an example of a gay person here, it can be any other identity we have of ourselves – straight person, doctor, roadsweeper, vegetarian, socialist, Buddhist – all these and thousands more are terms of identity.) But to return to Chris. He is a deeply spiritual being, and with all that being gay has brought to him (which included much suffering in his relationships in his family), he has turned to an ever-deepening awareness of his true identity and his capacity to love.

Some gay people are fired up, as a result of 'coming out', with a passion to remove social and cultural inequalities that repress and prohibit what is a hugely important part of self-identity. Some have become 'professional' gays, not just in terms of their social activism but in subsuming every aspect of their worldview and behaviour to being gay, and for a while my friend Chris fell into this way of being. Almost every conversation, social perspective and decision was taken in terms of being gay. 'I am gay' became a mantra by which he introduced himself in each encounter.

Recently I had the opportunity to spend some time with someone who is very famous and openly gay. His opening words to me were, 'Of course, you know I'm gay?' And I replied, 'Of course, you know you are not.' He just looked at me in stunned silence and then in discussion later I think he understood. For there is a paradox here. Coming to terms with our sexuality can be an immensely liberating experience, but it can also be a trap. It is necessary to have an identity to feel free in the world, but all the great spiritual traditions demand that this identity then be surrendered to be truly liberated. When we make a god of ourselves, we set ourselves against that which may be beyond ourselves. Accepting homosexuality sets the gay person free from the social stigmas and oppressions that veil it, but gay people are then still called to 'remember that liberation in the broadest possible sense ideally means developing a broader more inclusive vision' (Clarke, 1996). Gay liberation, indeed any sexual liberation, is therefore not an end in itself, but part of a process towards true liberation where we no longer identify ourselves with a limited part of who we are – we are far more than our sexuality. Being stuck in any one identity – 'I am a nurse', 'I am a mother', 'I am gay', 'I am straight' – brings us confidently into a sense of self, but it restricts us from moving into that which lies beyond the self. Jesus talked about not getting into heaven easily if you are rich – and if heaven is enlightenment, union with the divine, then while we are rich in self-identity and attached to these roles, then the spiritual path runs into the sand. The Prophet emphasised surrendering all aspects of the self to attain the divine. The Buddha encouraged complete disconnection from attachment to identity in order to attain Nirvana – the pure 'sky of mind' in which our consciousness has dropped all connections to identity, while remaining in identity in order to function and do good in the world.

My own teacher, Ram Dass, used to say, 'Nobody gets into heaven.' Just repeat that phrase to yourself. Nobody does indeed get into heaven (whatever you perceive that to be) . . . 'somebody' forever stays outside it while they are busy being somebody! If we are busy being a gay or straight 'somebody' or any other role 'somebody', we have not found true liberation but only a step along the way. Rest there as you will, yet there is yet more liberation if you will seek it, as there is for all of those who, having found a role, are willing to surrender it and go beyond. Frederick Perls, Gestalt psychologist wrote:

> *Many people dedicate their lives to actualize a concept of what they should be like, rather than to actualize themselves. This difference between self-actualizing and self image actualizing is very important. Most people only live for their image . . . they are so busy projecting themselves as a this or that.'*   Perls, 1969, cited in Rowan, 2001

The spiritual journey is to find our individuality and inhabit it, but then an ongoing maturation of that journey calls us to leave it behind, as the butterfly casts off the pupa. To do that is much scarier. Having made all those sacrifices along the hard road towards acknowledging being gay (and, indeed, whatever identity we choose to see ourselves as) to oneself and others, it seems a bit of a spiritual downer to now be asked for more. But more there is – to take a step into the void where all identity is left behind. Yet in that void we may find 'the real person, who is free to play games or not to play games and never has to play games' (Rowan, 2001). A sexual identity (indeed, any identity) can prove a catalyst for empowerment and bringing people together in greater connection and social action. But it goes further than that, beyond the Western obsession with sexual identity and gender differences, for it is said in the Indo-Tibetan Buddhist texts that an 'understanding of non-duality, of emptiness, brings about a greater compassion'. Seeing through identities, male, female, gay, straight, 'manifests itself in a kind of equanimity of compassionate action in regard to all creatures' (Edelstein, 2001). Finding an identity and then surrendering it thus breaks the pattern of disconnection from others, dissolving the distinctions between human beings that inhibit our capacity for compassion. Identity thereby ceases to be our master and becomes merely a role we have in the world to serve us.

For Levine and Levine (1995) relationships of all kinds are about the discovery of and falling into unconditional love – and this is, of itself, a sacred act. To do so is not just to embrace the beloved other person or ourselves; it is embracing the Beloved, the divine, the sacred love. Our relationships in all their shapes and forms can therefore be soul work. To say, 'I have no spiritual discipline' is therefore a contradiction in terms, for every relationship, and human encounter is pregnant with as much material for spiritual work as sitting in the presence of a saint in a monastery or a mystic in a retreat. Relationships are as valid a spiritual practice as any other, when we approach them consciously. Indeed, in the busy and increasingly non-religious world, they may be emerging as the main spiritual practice available to us.

RIGHT UNDER YOUR NOSE (2)

I have suggested in different chapters that spirituality is not just a private indulgence but goes further and is acted out in the world. As Steindl-Rast (1991) comments:

> Having discovered the Divine in the depths of his or her own soul, the adept must then find the Divine in all life. This is, in fact, the adept's principal obligation and responsibility. To put it differently, having drunk of the fountain of life, the adept must complete the spiritual opus and practice compassion on the basis of the recognition that everything participates in the universal field of the Divine.

Our work, if we approach it consciously, is also a milieu for the practice of compassion.

Each working moment can also be an opportunity for 'soul growth' just like our relationships. We may undertake specific spiritual practices (e.g. worship through prayer or practise meditation) but our everyday work is replete with spiritual potential too. It provides us with countless teachings each day about others and ourselves. It confronts us with endless challenges to care in settings and relationships that may be hostile to caring.

All the great spiritual traditions speak of the path of service. Pursuing the inner work to discover right relationship with ourselves and perhaps our God may become a kind of spiritual self-gratification if it does not manifest itself in the world in some way. Whether we adopt a theistic or atheistic worldview, the message is the same – deepen your understanding of yourself and your part in the scheme of things, but at some point integrate this and apply it in your life and work. Thus, the occupation of the carer can provide an ideal opportunity to bring more love and compassion into the world through the relief of suffering. And it is a compassion without attachment (Ram Dass & Bush, 1992; Longaker, 1998), a way of being in the world that does not exhaust us with the burden of caring for others, but which liberates us to care from a place of resting at home within ourselves.

Most carers, therefore, need not look to retreat into a monastery, give up work to head for the nearest war zone or sacrifice all to care for the dying in a third-world country. For some people, these will be right courses of action in their spiritual search, if only for a while. For most of us, however, all that we need may be right at our fingertips in the here and now – our relationships and our work.

I recall a nurse I met working in a hospice some years ago, who felt a sudden urge to go and work overseas with Mother Theresa. Somehow, what the Mother was doing seemed so much more important than her own routine existence as she saw it. She wrote to me:

> 'One of my patients died while I was off duty and the family came in to thank me. I thought 'Why? She was young, she had everything to live for, they should have been enraged with me at their loss.' But they just kept thanking me, saying how we didn't appreciate all that we had done, all the little kindnesses, the attention to their loved one in her last hours. It began to dawn on me, after they had left, how little I valued what I already do. How what to me had become commonplace and ordinary was hugely important to those who receive it. I don't know why we don't always value what we are doing already. Maybe it's the 'grass is always greener' thing.

Valuing our own work of caring and recognising its essentially sacred nature is perhaps the most important thing we can do towards restoring the sacred to caring. What we do is significant – it matters – and coming to accept this when we so often undervalue the contribution we make is part of the process of getting into right relationship. Our work provides us with the milieu for action in the world. Valuing it, being in right relationship with it, helps us toward right relationship with ourselves. The path of service, espoused throughout the ages as a holy path, is available to those of us who are carers right now, should we choose it. Nurses, doctors, therapists – anyone in caring work – is blessed, in that sense, by not having to go out and find work of compassionate service. We are in it already. All we have to do is approach it more consciously. Supported by, for example, our insight work of meditation, we become more able to step out of the endless drama of work and relationships and see them for what they truly are – calls to ever-greater awakening.

END PIECE

One day it was announced around the monastery that a young Buddhist monk had attained enlightenment. Greatly impressed by this news, several of the other monks hurried to speak to him.
'We've heard you're enlightened, is this indeed true?' they asked excitedly.
'Yes,' replied the monk.
'How do you feel now?' they enquired in wonder.
'As miserable as ever,' he said.

Buddhist traditional story

In the face of a world seemingly spiralling into ever-deeper environmental, health and political catastrophe, we could be forgiven for feeling hopeless and powerless. 'We all want to change the world', sang John Lennon, and when we feel we cannot it is understandable that we might retreat into cynicism, violence or chocolate.

Such a despairing view is reinforced if we believe that this reality is all there is and that human consciousness is solely the product of a bunch of neurones. As I have written earlier in this book, such a view was not shared by the ancients and nor is it shared by modern quantum physicists or those at the cutting edge of consciousness research. If consciousness is not located merely within the brain, then huge possibilities open to us in health care and beyond, such as the fascinating studies conducted on non-local healing. If individual and collective consciousness can influence, albeit subtly, physical reality, then there is no need to lapse into the depressing, 'There's nothing I can do.' For we can all do something; each small act by or upon ourselves may contribute to the whole, for the good of all.

Coelho (1993) reinforces this in his delightful modern fable where he writes: 'When we strive to become better than we are, everything around us becomes better too.' And Andrew Harvey (1991), documenting his remarkable spiritual awakening, says, 'No awakening can be personal or selfish. Every awakening spreads its power and light throughout the world.' If we cannot change the world, then we can at least change a little of ourselves – by working to be more compassionate, more open-hearted, more authentic – and thereby we might just affect the world as well. Like a pebble cast into a pool, the ripples of awareness in our own consciousness spread far and wide. Not all of us can protest at a G8 summit, but we can still act quietly and gently upon our own natures and work in small ways to affect our immediate community.

Consider the potential of those of us who work in health care – our numbers are huge. In the UK, for example, the NHS is the largest employer in the world after the army of the People's Republic of China. If even a small percentage of that workforce were to expand their consciousness with greater spiritual awakening, then the impact on ourselves and those we serve could be huge. Likewise, health services across the globe tend to employ very large numbers of people – and we are people who stand at the precipice of human suffering in all its forms for so many. We have the tools to hand – for best caring practice directly brings wellbeing for others into the world, not necessarily on a grand scale, but in the everyday acts of 'heroism' – the day-by-day and night-by-night attentions to the wellbeing of others, often in the face of considerable odds (Lanara, 1981).

Kornfield (2000) writes that:

> Sometimes it is necessary to march, sometimes it is necessary to sit, to pray. Each in turn can bring the heart and the world back to balance. For us to act wisely, our compassion must be balanced with equanimity, the ability to let things be as they are. Just as our passionate heart can be touched by the sorrows of the world, so too we must remember that it is not our responsibility to fix all the brokenness of the world – only to fix what we can.

In an holistic universe, the part affects the whole; every bit of 'fixing' thereby contributes to the whole. Hartmann (1997), too, picks up this theme, of how personal health, consciousness and behaviour are intimately linked to the same phenomena in the wider world. Thus, through a sensitive and gentle combination of being and doing, we can each play a part in dispersing the general and individual despair. We can affect the personal and collective zeitgeist that tells us that our bodies and minds are all that we are and that nothing can reach beyond these to transform the world we live in, seemingly hell-bent on oblivion.

In Kornfield's book there is a story of hope, illustrating that small acts are equally important as the grand gesture. An old man is walking along a beach, which is covered with enormous numbers of dying starfish, cast upon the sand by a spring storm. The old man is walking among the starfish, tossing them back into the waves one by one. A passing visitor looks surprised and asks him what he is doing. 'I'm trying to help this starfish,' replies the old man. 'But there are thousands here,' scoffs the sceptical visitor, 'Don't you realise that throwing back a handful doesn't matter?' 'Matters to this one,' the old man replies as he tosses one more starfish back into the ocean.

References

Abbot, N. C. (2000). Healing as a therapy for human disease: a systematic review. Journal of Alternative and Complementary Medicine 6 (2), 159-169.

Achterberg, J. (1990). Woman as Healer. Ryder, London.

Akinsanya, J. & Rouse, P. (1991). Who Will Care? A survey of the knowledge and attitudes of hospital nurses to people with HIV/AIDS. Anglia Polytechnic Faculty of Health and Social Work, Chelmsford.

Allen, R. (ed.) (1990). The Concise Oxford Dictionary. Clarendon, Oxford.

Anderson, S. (ed.) (1996). The Virago Book of Spirituality. Virago, London.

Anon. (1975). A Course in Miracles. Arkana, Harmondsworth.

Armstrong, K. (1993). A History of God. Ballantine, New York.

Armstrong, K. (2001). The Battle for God – fundamentalism in Judaism, Christianity and Islam. HarperCollins, London.

Artress, L. (1995). Walking a Sacred Path – rediscovering the labyrinth as a sacred tool. Riverhead, New York.

Attar, F. ud-din (1984). The Conference of the Birds. Darbandi, A. & Davis, D. (trans.). Penguin, Harmondsworth.

Babbs, J. (1991). New age fundamentalism. In: Zwieg, C. & Adams, J. (eds). Meeting the Shadow – the hidden power of the dark side of human nature. Putnam, New York.

Badiner, A. & Hunt, A. (eds). (2002). Zig Zag Zen. Chronicle, San Francisco.

Baldwin, J. (1985). Notes of a Native Son. PlutoPress, New York.

Barasch, M. (1993). The Healing Path. Arkana/Penguin, London.

Barker, P. & Buchanan-Barker, P. (2004). Spirituality and Mental Health Breakthrough. Whurr, London.

Barrett, D. (1996). Sects, Cults and Alternative Religions. Blandford, London.

Beddington-Behrens, S. (2001). A dangerous opportunity: the spiritual challenges of the events of September 11th. Network: the Scientific and Medical Network Review 77, 6-8.

Benn, C. (2000). Does faith contribute to healing? Scientific evidence for a correlation between spirituality and health. Sacred Space 1 (4), 7-13.

Benner, P. (1984). From Novice to Expert. Addison Wesley, New York.

Benner, P. & Wrubel, J. (1989). The Primacy of Caring. Addison Wesley, New York.

Bennett, O. (2003). Up where you belong. The Sunday Review, 5 January, 16-19.

Benson, H. (1996). Timeless Healing. Schuster, London.

Bible. (1999). New Revised Standard Version. Oxford University Press, Oxford.

Biley, F. & Wright, S. (1997). Towards a defence of nursing routine and ritual. Journal of Clinical Nursing 6, 115-119.

Blue, L. (2001). The Little Book of Blue Thoughts. Rider, London.

Bly, R. (1990). Iron John. Addison Wesley, Menlo Park.

Bly, R. (1991). The long bag we drag behind us. In: Zwieg, C. & Adams, J. (eds). Meeting the Shadow – the hidden power of the dark side of human nature. Putnam, New York.

Bohm, D. (1973). Quantum theory as an indication of a new order in physics; implicate and explicate order in physical law. Foundations of Physics 3, 139-168.

Borrill, C., Wall, T., West, M., Hardy, G. et al. (1998). Mental Health of the Workforce in NHS Trusts. Institute of Work Psychology, University of Sheffield, Sheffield.

Boux, D. (ed.) (1999) Woman – a unique tribute. Shepheard-Walwyn, London.

Brandon, D. (1986). Simply Meditate. Tao, Preston.

Braud, W. (2000). Wellness implications of retroactive intentional influence: exploring an outrageous hypothesis. Alternative Therapies in Health and Medicine 6 (1), 47-48.

Briskin, A. (1998). The Stirring of Soul in the Workplace. Berrett-Koehler, San Francisco.

British Medical Journal. (2001). Editorial – restoring the soul of medicine. BMJ 322 (7279), 113.

Brown, M. (1998). The Spiritual Tourist. Bloomsbury, London.

Buber, M. (1937). I and Thou. Clark, Edinburgh.

Burkhardt, M.A. & Jacobsen, M.G.N. (2000). Spirituality and health. In: Dossey, B.M., Keegan, L. & Guzetta, C. (eds). Holistic Nursing – a handbook for practice. Aspen, Gaithersburg.

Butler, A. (1968). Hippocratic Oath. New England Journal of Medicine 278, 48-49.

Byrd, R. (1988). Positive therapeutic effects of intercessionary prayer in a coronary care unit population. Southern Medical Journal 81 (7), 826-829.

Calhoun, C. (1995). Standing for something. Journal of Philosophy 92 (5), 235-260.

Campbell, A. (1984). Moderated Love. SPCK, London.

Caplan, M. (1999). Halfway Up the Mountain. Hohm, Prescott.

Caplan, M. (2002). Do You Need a Guru? Thorsons, London.

Cha, K., Wirth, D. & Lobo, R. (2001). Does prayer influence the success of in vitro fertilization-embryo transfer? Report of a masked randomized trial. Journal of Reproductive Medicine 46 (9), 781-787.

Charman, R.A. (2000). Placing healers, healees, and healing into a wider research context. Journal of Alternative and Complementary Medicine 6 (2), 177-180.

Chittick, W. (1983). The Sufi Path of Love: the spiritual teachings of Rumi. Suny, Albany.

Chopra, D. (1996). The Seven Spiritual Laws of Success. Bantam, London.

Clarke, J.M. (1996). Gay Spirituality. In: van Ness, P. (ed.) Spirituality and the Secular Quest. SCM, London.

Cobell, D. (2002). Losing my religion. Nursing Standard 16 (20), 20-21.

Coelho, P. (1993). The Alchemist. HarperCollins, London.

Confederation of British Industry. (1999). Promoting Mental Health at Work. Confederation of British Industry, London.

Cope, J. (1998). The Modern Antiquarian. Thorsons, London.

Dalrymple, T. (2000). Our lives in their hands. The Guardian, 2 February, 2-3.

Davies, N. (1993). Murder on Ward 4. Chatto and Windus, London.

Davies, O. (trans.) (1994). Meister Eckhart – selected writings. Penguin, Harmondsworth.

Dawood, N. (trans.) Qur'an. (1991). Penguin, Harmondsworth.

Deikman, A. (1990). The Wrong Way Home – uncovering patterns of cult behavior in American society. Beacon, Boston.

Department of Health. (2004). NHS Chaplaincy – meeting the religious and spiritual needs of patients and staff. Department of Health, London.

Dionysius the Areopagite. (1920). On the Divine Names and the Mystical Theology. Rolt, C. (trans.). Methuen, London.

Dossey, B. (1999). Florence Nightingale: mystic, visionary, healer. Springhouse, Springhouse PA.

Dossey, B. (2001). A Conversation with Barbara Dossey. Sacred Space 2 (3), 19-32.

Dossey, L. (1996). Prayer is Good Medicine. HarperCollins, San Francisco.

Dossey, L. (1997a). Healing Words. HarperCollins, New York.

Dossey, L. (1997b). The forces of healing; reflections on energy, consciousness and the beef stroganoff principle. Alternative Therapies in Health and Medicine 3 (5), 8-14.

Dossey, L. (1999). Do religion and spirituality matter in health? A response to the recent article in The Lancet. Alternative Therapies 5 (3), 16-18.

Dossey, L. (2001). Consciousness, spirituality and healing. Sacred Space 2 (4), 8-12.

Dostoyevsky, F. (1880). The Brothers Karamazov. Penguin, Harmondsworth (reprint 1993).

Douglas-Klotz, N. (1999). The Hidden Gospel. Quest, Wheaton.

Doyle, B. (1983). Meditations with Julian of Norwich. Bear, Santa Fe.

Duffin, C. (2003). Looking at alternatives. Nursing Standard 17 (33), 12-13.

Easwaran, E. (trans.) (1988). The Upanishads. Arkana, London.

Edelstein, A. (2001). An interview with Jose Cabazon. What is enlightenment? 20 (Fall), 137-215.

Eliot, T.S. (1944). The Four Quartets. Harcourt Brace Jovanovich, London.

Engel, J.D., Pethtel, L., Ways, P. & Zarconi, J. (2000). The spiritual dimension in the physician-patient relationship. Sacred Space 1 (3), 4-11.

Faugier, J. & Hicken, D. (1996). AIDS and HIV, the Nursing Response. Chapman Hall, London.

Feinstein, A.R. & Horwitz, R.L. (1997). Problems in the 'evidence' of evidence-based medicine. American Journal of Medicine 103, 529-535.

Ford, P. & Walsh, M. (1994). New Rituals for Old. Butterworth Heinemann, London.

Forder, J. & Forder, E. (eds) (1995). The Light Within. Usha, Cumbria.

Foundation for Integrated Health. (2003). Setting the Agenda for the Future. The Prince of Wales Foundation for Integrated Health, London.

Foundation for Integrated Medicine. (2003). A Guide to Our Work. Foundation for Integrated Medicine, London.

Frank, A. (1991). At the Will of the Body – reflections on illness. Houghton Mifflin, New York.

Friedlander, S. (2003). Rumi and the Whirling Dervishes. Parabola, New York.

Fry, C. (1951). A Sleep of Prisoners. Oxford University Press, Oxford.

Fulder, S. (1996). The Handbook of Alternative and Complementary Medicine. Oxford University Press, Oxford.

Gandhi, M.K. (1924). Cited on Gandhi website: www.mkgandhi.org.

Gardner, H. (ed.) (1989). The New Oxford Book of English Verse. Oxford University Press, Oxford.

Gibran, K. (1933). The Garden of the Prophet. Penguin, Harmondsworth.

Glouberman, D. (2002). The Joy of Burnout; how the end of the world can be a new beginning. Hodder Mobius, London.

Goldhagen, D. (1997). Hitler's Willing Executioners. Abacus, London.

Goleman, D. (1995). Emotional Intelligence. Bantam, New York.

Gordon, P. (1998). Secular thoughts. The Guardian, Society, 30 December, 18-19.

Gordon, S. (1997). Life Support – three nurses on the front line. Little Brown, New York.

Graham, H. (1999). Complementary Therapies in Context: the psychology of healing. Kingsley, London.

Green, C.A. (1998). Reflection on a therapeutic touch experience: case study 2. Complementary Therapies in Nursing and Midwifery 4, 17-21.

Gregory of Nyasa. (1993). On the Soul and the Resurrection. Roth, C. (trans.). St Valdimir's Seminary Press, New York.

Griffith, J. (2002). Encountering the Sacred in Psychotherapy. Guildford, London.

Grof, S. (1980). LSD Psychotherapy. Hunter, Almeda.

Guenther, M. (2002). Holy Listening. DLT, London.

Hacker, G. (1998). The Healing Stream. Darton, Longman and Todd, London.

Hafiz. (1996). I Heard God Laughing – renderings of Hafiz. Ladinsky, D. (trans.). Sufism Reoriented, Walnut Creek.

Halevi, Y. (2002). Poems from the Divan. Levin, G. (trans.). Anvil, London.

Hamer, D. (2004). The God Gene: How faith is hard-wired into our genes. Doubleday, London.

Hammer, M., Nichols, D. & Armstrong, L. (1992). A ritual rememberance. American Journal of Maternal Child Nursing 17, 310-313.

Harrison, S. (2003). Soul survivors. Nursing Standard 17 (35), 16-17.

Hartmann, T. (1997). The Prophet's Way. Mythical Books, Northfield.

Harvey, A. (1991). Hidden Journey. Rider, London.

Hatfield, D. (1999). Gallup Organisation: new research links emotional intelligence with profitability. The Inner Edge 1(5), 5-9.

Hay, D. (2004). Spirituality as a human universal; the empirical evidence. Spirituality and Health conference, University of Aberdeen, January 2003 (unpublished paper).

Hay, D. & Hunt, K. (2000). The spirituality of people who don't go to church; final report. Adult Spirituality Project, Nottingham University, Nottingham.

Hawkins, P. & Shohet, R. (1991). Supervision in the Helping Professions. Open University Press, Milton Keynes.

Health Education Authority. (1996). Organisational Stress. Health Education Authority, London.

Health Education Authority. (1998). More Than Brown Bread and Aerobics. Health Education Authority, London.

Health and Safety Executive. (2004). Data taken from website January 2004: www.hse.gov.uk/statistics/pdf/swi04.pdf

Hegel, G.W.F. (1892). The Lesser Logic. Wallace, W. (ed.). Clarendon, Oxford.

Hillman, J. (1979). The Dream of the Underworld. Harper and Row, New York.

Hodges, R.D. & Scofield, A.M. (1995). Is spiritual healing a valid and effective therapy? Journal of the Royal Society of Medicine 88, 203-207.

Hodgkin, P. (1996). Medicine, postmodernism and the end of certainty. British Medical Journal 313, 1568-1569.

Holden, M. (2002a). Boundless Love. Rider, London.

Holden, M. (2002b). A Conversation with Miranda Holden. Sacred Space 3 (3), 16-23.

Holdom, K. (1999). Whose idea was this? The Guardian, 20 May, 8.

Holland, C. (1993). An ethnographic study of nursing culture as an exploration for determining the existence of a system of ritual. Journal of Advanced Nursing 18, 1461-1470.

Hudson, R. (2003). The spirit of the age and the spirit of ageing. Sacred Space 4 (1), 5-11.

Hugman, R. (1991). Power in Caring Professions. Macmillan, London.

Huxley, A. (1954). The Doors of Perception. HarperCollins, London (reprint 1994).

Ibn Al-'Arabi. (1980). The Bezels of Wisdom. Austin, R. (trans.). Paulist, Mahwah.

Jesse, R. (2002). A survey of the entheogens. In: Badiner, A. & Hunt, A. (eds) Zig Zag Zen. Chronicle, San Francisco.

Jones, J. (1996). In the Middle of this Road We Call Our Life. HarperCollins, London.

Jung, C. (1961). Modern Man in Search of Soul. Routledge & Kegan Paul, London.

Kabat-Zinn, J. (1996). Full Catastrophe Living. Piatkus, London.

Kafka, F. (1916). Metamorphosis. Penguin, London (reprint 1974).

Kelting, T. (1995). The nature of nature. Parabola 20 (1), 24-26.

Kimble, M. (2001). Beyond the biomedical paradigm: generating a spiritual vision of ageing. Journal of Religious Gerontology 12 (3/4), 31-41.

Kornfield, J. (2000). After the Ecstasy, the Laundry. Rider, London.

Krucoff, M., Crater, S., Green, C., Maas, A., Sekevitch, J., Lane, J., Loeffler, K., Morris, K., Bashore, T. & Koenig, H. (2001). Integrative noetic therapies as adjuncts to percutaneous intervention during unstable coronary syndromes: monitoring and actualization of noetic training (MANTRA) feasability pilot. American Heart Journal 142 (5), 760-767.

Kubler-Ross, E. (1969). On Death and Dying. Macmillan, New York.

Lanara, V. (1981). Heroism as a Nursing Value. Sisterhood Evniki, Athens.

Le Shan, L. (1974). How to Meditate. HarperCollins, London.

Lee, D. (2001). The morning tea break ritual: a case study. International Journal of Nursing Practice 7, 69-73.

Lee, Peggy. (1969). Is That All There Is? Columbia Records.

Leibovici, L. (2001). The effects of remote, retroactive intercessionary prayer on outcomes in patients with bloodstream infection: randomised controlled trial. British Medical Journal 323, 1450-1451.

Lerner, M. (2000). Spirit Matters. Hampton Roads, Charlottesville.

Levine, S. & Levine, O. (1995). Embracing the Beloved. Doubleday, New York.

Lewis, D. (1999). A survey of therapeutic touch practitioners. Nursing Standard 13 (30), 27-29.

Lifton, R. (1986). The Nazi Doctors. Papermac, London.

Longaker, C. (1998). Facing Death and Finding Hope. Arrow, London.

Lott, T. (2004). The Scent of Dried Roses. Penguin, London.

Macrae, J. (1995). Nightingale's spiritual philosophy and its significance for modern nursing. Image – Journal of Nursing Scholarship 27 (1), 8-10.

Maimonides. (1952). The Guide for the Perplexed. Rabin, C. (trans.). Hackett, Cambridge.

Main, J. (1988). The Inner Christ. DLT, London.

Mann, A. (1993). Sacred Architecture. Element, Shaftesbury.

Martin, J. (1984). Hospitals in Trouble. Blackwell, Oxford.

Mascaro, J. (trans.) (1962). The Bhagavad Gita. Penguin, Harmondsworth.

Mascaro, J. (trans.) (1973). The Dhammapada. Penguin, Harmondsworth.

Maxwell, M. & Tschudin, V. (1996). Seeing the Invisible. Arkana, London.

McMann, J. (1998). Altars and Icons – sacred spaces in everyday lives. Chronicle, San Francisco.

McSherry, W. (2000). Making Sense of Spirituality in Nursing Practice. Churchill Livingstone, Edinburgh.

Milne, A.A. (1982). Winnie the Pooh and the House at Pooh Corner. Methuen, London (reprint).

Mitchell, J. (1976). Song for Sharon. On: Hejira. Elektra/Asylum Records, New York.

MORI Social Research Institute. (2003). Heaven and Earth Survey – three in five believe in God. MORI, London: www.mori.com/polls/2003/bbc-heavenandearth.shtml

Muller, W. (1999). Sabbath: restoring the sacred rhythm of rest. Bantam, New York.

Nathan, M. (2000). A study of patients' perceptions and views on spiritual care in mental health practice. Sacred Space 2 (2), 18-24 and 2 (4), 33-41 (parts 1 and 2 respectively).

NHS England. (2003). NHS chaplaincy; meeting the religious and spiritual needs of patients and staff. Department of Health, London.

NHS Scotland. (2002). Guidelines on chaplaincy and spiritual care in the NHS in Scotland. National Health Service HDL-2002-76.

National Research Register. (2002). Department of Health, 22 August 2002: www.Update-software.com/National/about-norr.html

Newberg, A., D'Aquili, E. & Rause, V. (2001). Why God Won't Go Away. Ballantine, New York.

Newman, M. (1986). Health as Expanding Consciousness. Mosby, St Louis.

Nietzsche, F. (1974). The Gay Science. Kaufmann, W. (trans.). Vintage, New York.

Nightingale, F. (1869). Notes on Nursing; what it is and what it is not. Churchill Livingstone, Edinburgh.

Nouwen, H. (1997). The Inner Voice of Love. DLT, London.

O'Brien, M. (1982). The need for spiritual integrity in human needs and the nursing process. In: Yura, H. & Walsh, M. (eds). The Nursing Process. Appleton-Century-Crofts, New York.

Olsen, D.T. (1999). The concept of holiness. In: O'Day, G. & Peterson, D. (eds). The Access Bible. Oxford University Press, Oxford.

Oxford English Dictionary. (1999). Clarendon, Oxford.

Palmer, M. & Palmer, N. (1997). Sacred Britain. Piatkus, London.

Parsons, S. (2000). Ungodly Fear. Lion, Oxford.

Pert, C. (1997). Molecules of Emotion. Scribner, New York.

Peters, D. (ed.) (2002). Understanding the Placebo Effect in Complementary Medicine – theory, practice and research. Churchill Livingstone, Edinburgh.

Pierpoint, I. (2001). The Vegas Study. Business Research International, London.

Pierrakos, E. & Saly, J. (1993). Creating Union – the pathwork of relationship. Pathwork Press, Madison.

Pinchbeck, D. (2003). Breaking Open the Head. Flamingo, London.

Pinney, R. (1981). Creative Listening (personal publication – cited in Pym op. cit.)

Plato. (1987). The Republic. Reed, D. (trans.). Penguin, London.

Porter, A. (2002). The interfaith seminary – a closer look at grace. Sacred Space 3 (2), 13-15.

Prigogine, I. & Stenders, I. (1984). Order Out of Chaos. Bantam, New York.

Puchalski, C. (2004). Conversation. Spirituality and Health International 5 (2), 82-87.

Pym, J. (1999). Listening to the Light. Rider, London.

Quinn, J.F. & Strelkauskas, A.J. (1993). Psychoimmunologic effects of therapeutic touch on practitioners and recently bereaved recipients: a pilot study. Advances in Nursing Science 15 (4), 13-26.

Ram Dass. (1971). Be Here Now. Crown, New York.

Ram Dass. (1997). The Book of Grace: a series of tape recordings of Ram Dass' teachings. Seva Foundation, San Francisco.

Ram Dass. (2000). Still Here. Hodder and Stoughton, London.

Ram Dass. (2002). One liners – a mini manual for the spiritual life. Bell Tower, New York.

Ram Dass & Bush, M. (1992). Compassion in Action. Bell Tower, New York.

Ram Dass & Gorman, P. (1990). How Can I Help? Knopf, New York.

Ray, P.H. (1996). The integral culture survey – a study of the emergence of transformational values in America. Institute of Noetic Sciences, Sausalito.

Rayes-Hughes, A. (2000). Nursing the Iraqi Leader. Nursing Times 96 (41), 20.

Reilly, D. (2001). Enhancing human healing. British Medical Journal 322 (7279), 120-121.

Reoch, R. (2001). Are we up to death? Raft 19 (Spring), 33-34.

Rilke, R.M. (1981). Selected Poems. Bly, R. (trans.). Harper and Row, London.

Roemischer, J. (2003). Traditions on the edge – can the past meet the future? What is Enlightenment 23 (Spring/Summer), 56-68.

Rogers, M. (1970). An Introduction to the Theoretical Basis of Nursing. Davies, Philadelphia.

Rogers, M. (1990). Nursing science of unitary, irreducible, human beings; update 1990. In: Barrett, E. (ed.). Visions of Rogers' Science-based Nursing. National League for Nursing, New York.

Ross, H. (1998). Jesus Untouched by the Church – his teachings in the gospel of St Thomas. Ebor, York.

Rowan, J. (2001). Ordinary Ecstasy. Brunner Routledge, Hove.

Rumi, J. (1997). The Illuminated Rumi. Barks, C. (trans.). Broadway, New York.

Sahajananda, J. (2003). You are the Light – rediscovering the Eastern Jesus. O Books, Alresford.

St John of the Cross. (1973). The Dark Night of the Soul. Zimmerman, B. (trans.). Clarke, Cambridge.

St Theresa of Avila. (1995). The Interior Castle. van de Weyer, R. (trans.). HarperCollins, London.

Santorelli, S. (1999). Heal Thy Self: lessons on mindfulness in medicine. Random House, New York.

Saxby, J. (1983a). Jane Saxby. In: Jones, B. (ed.) Three Lives. NFCO, London.

Saxby, J. (1983b). (Private correspondence).

Sayre-Adams, J. & Wright, S.G. (2001). Therapeutic Touch. Churchill Livingstone, Edinburgh.

Schreoder-Sheker, T. (1994). Music for the dying: a personal account of the new field of music thanatology. Journal of Holistic Nursing 12 (1), 56-64.

Schultes, R.E. & Hofmann, A. (1992). Plants of the Gods. Healing Arts Press, Rochester.

Schumacher, E. (1977). A Guide for the Perplexed. Abacus, London.

Scott Peck, F. (1996). In Search of Stones. Hyperion, New York.

Segal, Z., Williams, J. & Teasdale, J. (2002). Mindfulness-based Cognitive Therapy for Depression. Guilford, New York.

Self, M. (2001). From Medicine to Miracle. HarperCollins, London.

Shakespeare, W. (1982). The Illustrated Shakespeare. Chancellor, London.

Skolimowski, H. (1992). Living Philosophy: ecophilosophy as a tree of life. Arkana, London.

Sloan, R., Bagiella, E. & Powell, T. (1999). Religion, spirituality and medicine. Lancet 353 (9153), 664-667.

Smith, H. (1964). Do drugs have religious import? American Journal of Philosophy 61 (18), 116-139.

Snow, C. & Willard, P. (1989). I'm Dying to Take Care of You. Professional Counsellor Books, Redmond.

Sogyal Rinpoche. (1992). The Tibetan Book of Living and Dying. Ryder, London.

Spears, L.C. (ed.) (1998). Insights on Leadership – service, stewardship, spirit and servant leadership. Wiley, London.

Sri Aurobindo. (1970). The Life Divine. Sri Aurobindo Ashram, Pondicherry.

Steindl-Rast, D. (1991). The shadow in Christianity. In: Zweig, C. & Abrams, J. (eds). Meeting the Shadow – the hidden power of the dark side of human nature. Putnam, New York.

Stone, V. (2000). Designing environments to nurture the spirit. Sacred Space 1 (4), 39-46.

Storr, A. (1996). Feet of Clay – a study of gurus. HarperCollins, London.

Stoter, D. (1995). Spiritual Aspects of Health Care. Mosby, London.

Streep, P. (trans.) (1994) Tao Te Ching. Bullfinch, London.

Tacey, D. (2003). The Spiritual Revolution. Harpercollins, Sydney.

Teasdale, W. (2001). The Mystic Heart. New World, Novato.

Thich Nhat Hanh. (1993). Present Moment; Wonderful Moment. Rider, London.

Thomas, R. (1999). The I society. The Guardian (Archive), 17 September.

Thorsons. (1999). The Way Ahead – Thorsons market research. Thorsons, London.

Underhill, E. (1993). Mysticism. Oneworld, Oxford (first published 1910).

Union of Liberal and Progressive Synagogues. (1995). Siddur Lev Chadash – services and prayers. ULPS, London.

Vardy, P. (1992). The Puzzle of Evil. Fount, London.

Vaughan, F. (1995). Shadows of the Sacred. Quest, Wheaton.

Vaughan, F. & Walsh, R. (1988). Gifts from a Course in Miracles. Tarcher/Putnam, New York.

Wakeman, H. (2002). Circles of Stillness – thoughts on contemplative prayer from the Julian meetings. Darton Longman Todd, London.

Walker, B. (1985). The Crone – woman of age, wisdom and power. Harper, San Francisco.

Walsch, N.M. (1995). Conversations with God – an uncommon dialogue. Hodder and Stoughton, London.

Walsh, M. & Ford, P. (1989). Nursing Rituals: research and rational actions. Heinemann, London.

Walsh, R. (2002). Mysticism: contemplative and chemical. In: Badiner, A. & Hunt, A. (eds). Zig Zag Zen. Chronicle, San Francisco.

Watson, L. (1980). Lifetide. Bantam, London.

Webb, T. (ed.) (1991). W.B. Yeats – selected poetry. Penguin, Harmondsworth.

Wheaton, K. (1987). Spain. APA, London.

Wilber, K. (1991). Taking responsibility for your shadow. In: Zwieg, C. & Adams, J. (eds). Meeting the Shadow – the hidden power of the dark side of human nature. Putnam, New York.

Wilber, K. (1998). The Essential Wilber: an introductory reader. Shambala, Boston.

Williams, S., Mitchie, S. & Pattani, S. (1998). Improving the Health of the NHS Workforce. Nuffield, London.

Witteveen, H. (1997). Universal Sufism. Element, Shaftesbury.

Wolters, C. (trans., author anon.) (1978). The Cloud of Unknowing. Penguin, Harmondsworth.

Wolterstorff, N. (1987). Lament for a Son. Eerdmans, Grand Rapids.

Woodham, A. & Peters, D. (1997). The Encyclopaedia of Complementary Medicine. Dorling Kindersley, London.

Woodman, M. & Dickson, E. (1996). Dancing in the Flames – the dark goddess in the transformation of consciousness. Gill and Macmillan, Dublin.

World Health Organization. (1994). Guidelines for the Primary Prevention of Mental, Neurological and Psychosocial Disorders 5 – Staff Burnout. World Health Organization Division of Mental Health No. who/mnh/mnd/94.21, Geneva.

Wright, S.G. (2004a). The Bristol approach. Nursing Standard 18 (36), 16-19.

Wright, S.G. (2004b). Is there no alternative? Nursing Standard 18 (41), 14-15.

Wright, S.G. & Sayre-Adams, J. (2000). Sacred Space – right relationship and spirituality in health care. Churchill Livingstone, London.

Wright, S., Gough, P. & Poulton, B. (1998). Imagining the Future (full report). Royal College of Nursing, London.

Young-Eisendrath, P. & Miller, M. (2000). The Psychology of Mature Spirituality. Routledge, London.

Zohar, D. & Marshall, I. (2000). Spiritual Intelligence – the ultimate intelligence. Bloomsbury, London.

Zwieg, C. & Adams, J. (eds). (1991). Meeting the Shadow – the hidden power of the dark side of human nature. Putnam, New York.

Index